Handbook of
Obstetric Medicine

Catherine Nelson-Piercy
Consultant Obstetric Physician
Guy's & St Thomas' Hospital Trust
and Whipps Cross Hospital, London, UK

MARTIN DUNITZ

© 1997, 2002 Martin Dunitz Ltd, a member of the Taylor & Francis group

First edition published in the United Kingdom in 1997
by Isis Medical Media Ltd, 58 St Aldgates, Oxford OX1 1ST

Second edition published in the United Kingdom in 2002
by Martin Dunitz Ltd, The Livery House, 7–9 Pratt Street, London NW1 0AE
Tel.: +44 (0) 20 74822202
Fax.: +44 (0) 20 72670159
E-mail: info.@dunitz.co.uk
Website: http://www.dunitz.co.uk

Although every effort has been made to ensure that all owners of copyright material have been
acknowledged in this publication, we would be glad to acknowledge in subsequent reprints or
editions any omissions brought to our attention.

The Author has asserted her right under the Copyright, Designs and Patents Act 1988 to be identified
as the Author of this Work.
Although every effort has been made to ensure that drug doses and other information are presented
accurately in this publication, the ultimate responsibility rests with the prescribing physician. Neither
the publishers nor the authors can be held responsible for errors or for any consequences arising
from the use of information contained herein. For detailed prescribing information or instructions
on the use of any product or procedure discussed herein, please consult the prescribing information
or instructional material issued by the manufacturer.

A CIP record for this book is available from the British Library.

ISBN 1 1-84184-118-8

Distributed in the USA by
Fulfilment Center
Taylor & Francis
7625 Empire Drive
Florence, KY 41042, USA
Toll Free Tel.: +1 800 634 7064
E-mail: cserve@routledge_ny.com

Distributed in Canada by
Taylor & Francis
74 Rolark Drive
Scarborough, Ontario M1R 4G2, Canada
Toll Free Tel.: +1 877 226 2237
E-mail: tal_fran@istar.ca

Distributed in the rest of the world by
ITPS Limited
Cheriton House
North Way
Andover, Hampshire SP10 5BE, UK
Tel.: +44 (0)1264 332424
E-mail: reception@itps.co.uk

Composition by Wearset Ltd, Boldon, Tyne and Wear
Printed and bound in Spain

Contents

Foreword to the first edition

Obstetric medicine is becoming increasingly important for obstetricians: more 'normal' pregnancies are being looked after by midwives, leaving only complicated pregnancies for the obstetrician. About half of these pregnancies are abnormal because of fetal factors, such as intra-uterine growth retardation, or strictly obstetric factors, for example breech presentation. The remainder are abnormal because of medical matters. Obstetricians of the future will have to take more responsibility for the medical problems of pregnancy.

Obstetric medicine is not well covered in traditional textbooks of obstetrics at undergraduate or postgraduate level. This handbook, therefore, fills a very important gap. It is remarkably comprehensive and yet easily referred to in an emergency. Particularly helpful is the second section directed towards presenting symptoms such as breathlessness, chest pain and headache. If a doctor does not know that headache can be a presenting symptom of cerebral vein thrombosis, he or she is unlikely to read the relevant section of the thromboembolic disease chapter.

Catherine Nelson-Piercy is well qualified to write this text. She is one of the very few Consultant Physicians to hold appointments in obstetric medicine. Her broad training has given her first-hand experience of even the less common medical complications of pregnancy that are described so well in this text. I am confident that the book will become a standard reference for all clinicans caring for pregnant women.

Michael de Swiet
Consultant Physician
Queen Charlotte's and Chelsea Hospital
London, UK

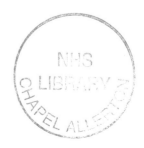

Preface to the first edition

Care of the pregnant woman with a medical condition requires knowledge of how the disease may be affected by pregnancy and vice versa. Concern for the welfare of the fetus may influence management and particularly the choice of drugs. Many physicians are unfamiliar with the physiological adaptation to pregnancy and the medical disorders that may be encountered in obstetric practice. There exists an understandable reluctance to institute investigations and therapies with which physicians are very experienced in the non-pregnant patient. Similarly, since many medical conditions are seen infrequently in general obstetric practice, obstetricians may not feel confident to manage all medical complications of pregnancy.

The field of obstetric medicine is vast since virtually any medical condition may complicate pregnancy. Certain diseases, more common in women of child-bearing age, are encountered more frequently in obstetric practice. Medical disorders complicating pregnancy may pre-date, coincide with or be specific to pregnancy. As the body of scientific knowledge grows and we understand more about conditions such as pre-eclampsia and intrahepatic cholestasis of pregnancy, the speciality of obstetric medicine continues to develop.

The aim of this handbook is to provide a practical guide for general practitioners, obstetricians and physicians of all grades who care for pregnant women with medical problems. It is not comprehensive, but highlights the most important and relevant factors in the management of medical complications in pregnancy. The opinions contained within the text are as far as possible a synthesis of contemporary literature review, established practice and evidence-based medicine. Inevitably, personal preference has influenced certain recommendations.

The chapters are organised by system in Section A and cover the most common and important medical conditions encountered in pregnancy. This is followed by Section B, providing a practical, problem-based approach to common symptoms, signs and biochemical abnormalities encountered in pregnancy, the emphasis being on differential diagnosis.

I am indebted to Dr Michael de Swiet for encouraging and supporting my decision to become an obstetric physician, for teaching me and allowing me to share his wealth of experience. My thanks also to Professor John Lumley and Dr Susan Bewley, without whose help and encouragement this book would never have reached fruition, and the many senior and junior doctors who provided valuable comments.

I hope this handbook proves a useful manual for practising obstetricians who may not have access to an obstetric physician, and for physicians who may be uneasy, as I once was, about being called to see a pregnant woman with an acute medical problem.

Preface to the second edition

Many fields within obstetric medicine have progressed rapidly since the first edition of this handbook: basic scientific as well as clinical research continue to improve our understanding of pregnancy-specific disorders, such as pre-eclampsia and obstetric cholestasis.

In preparing this second edition I have taken note of the many helpful comments from readers. The basic chapter format within Section A is maintained with bullet points covering pathophysiology, the interactions between the medical conditions and pregnancy and 'points to remember' boxes. All chapters have been substantially updated together with contemporary suggestions for further reading. New sections covering rare but important conditions such as myotonic dystrophy, Ehlers–Danlos syndrome, pregnancy-associated osteoporosis and pre-existing liver disease have been added. Rapid advances in HIV and thrombophilia are reflected in extensive revision to these chapters.

Section B, focusing on differential diagnosis, retains the original format but has been updated. I have included an appendix of normal values in pregnancy/non-pregnancy as a 'ready reference' and an appendix summarising drugs to be avoided in pregnancy, with cross-reference to more detailed discussion elsewhere in the *Handbook*.

Encouragement from colleagues, trainees in obstetrics, and midwives who have found the *Handbook* useful has made the task of writing the second edition enjoyable. I would in particular like to acknowledge the help and invaluable comments and suggestions of Dr Hassan Shehata.

I hope this volume continues to motivate health care professionals to further their understanding of obstetric medicine and provide appropriate care for pregnant women with medical problems.

Glossary

ABG	Arterial blood gases
aCL	Anticardiolipin antibodies
ACTH	Adrenocorticotrophic hormone
AFLP	Acute fatty liver of pregnancy
ALP	Alkaline phosphatase
ANA	Anti-nuclear antibodies
APS	Antiphospholipid syndrome
CMV	Cytomegalovirus
CSF	Cerebrospinal fluid
CT	Computerised tomography
CTG	Cardiotocography
CVP	Central venous pressure
CXR	Chest X-ray
DIC	Disseminated intravascular coagulation
EBV	Epstein–Barr virus
ECG	Electrocardiogram
EEG	Electroencephalogram
FBC	Full blood count
FEV_1	Forced expiratory volume in 1 second
FFP	Fresh frozen plasma
GH	Growth hormone
HELLP	Haemolysis, Elevated Liver enzymes, and Low Platelets (syndrome)
HPL	Human placental lactogen
HUS	Haemolytic uraemic syndrome
HVS	High vaginal swab
IGT	Impaired glucose tolerance
IUGR	Intrauterine growth retardation
LFTs	Liver function tests
LMP	Last menstrual period

LSCS	Lower segment caesarean section
MAP	Mean arterial (blood) pressure = D + 1/3 (S-D), where D = diastolic blood pressure and S = systolic blood pressure
MgSO$_4$	Magnesium sulphate
MRI	Magnetic resonance imaging
MSU	Mid-stream urine specimen
OGTT	Oral glucose tolerance test
PEFR	Peak expiratory flow rate
PNMR	Perinatal mortality rate
RDS	Respiratory distress syndrome
SLE	Systemic lupus erythematosus
SVD	Spontaneous vaginal delivery
SVR	Systemic vascular resistance
TFTs	Thyroid function tests
TSH	Thyroid-stimulating hormone
TTP	Thrombotic thrombocytopenic purpura
U+E	Urea and electrolytes
US	Ultrasound
UTI	Urinary tract infection
VMA	Vanillylmandelic acid
VSD	Ventricular septal defect
WBC	White blood cell
ZIG	Zoster immunoglobulin

To Sophie, Emma, Rebecca and Alice

SECTION A
Systems

CHAPTER 1

Hypertension and pre-eclampsia

Physiological changes	Risk factors
Scope of the problem	Diagnosis
Clinical features	Management
Pathogenesis	Prophylaxis
Recurrence/pre-pregnancy counselling	

Physiological changes

- Blood pressure is directly proportional to systemic vascular resistance and cardiac output.

- Vasodilation is probably the primary change in the circulation in pregnancy (see also Cardiovascular adaptation to pregnancy, p. 22).

- Before the increase in cardiac output can adequately compensate for the fall in systemic vascular resistance, blood pressure begins to decrease in early pregnancy. It continues to decrease in the second trimester of normal pregnancy until the nadir in systolic and diastolic blood pressure is reached by about 22–24 weeks' gestation. From then on, there is a steady rise to pre-pregnant levels until term.

- Phase V (disappearance) rather than phase IV (muffling) of Korotkoff sounds should be taken as the diastolic reading. Phase V is more reproducible, correlates better with intra-arterial measurements of diastolic blood pressure, and is more closely related to outcome.

- Blood pressure taken supine during the late second and third trimesters will be lower due to decreased venous return to the heart because of pressure from the gravid uterus. Blood pressure should be taken with the woman sitting or lying on her side with a 30° tilt. The upper arm (when using a cuff) should be at the same level as the heart.

- Blood pressure usually falls immediately after delivery, although tends to rise subsequently reaching a peak 3–4 days postpartum.

- A considerable number of previously normotensive women may become transiently hypertensive following delivery. This may relate to return of normal vascular tone and a period of vasomotor instability while normal, non-pregnant vasoregulation is re-established.

Scope of the problem

- Hypertension is the commonest medical problem encountered in pregnancy.
- It complicates 10–15% of all pregnancies. Mild pre-eclampsia affects up to 10% of primiparous women; the incidence of severe pre-eclampsia is about 1%.
- Eclampsia complicates about 1 in 2000 (0.05%) pregnancies in the UK and Europe. In some developing countries, the incidence reaches 1%.
- Eclampsia occurs in about 1–2% of women with pre-eclampsia in developed countries.
- Hypertensive disorders of pregnancy are a leading cause of maternal mortality in the UK; between seven and nine women die each year in the UK from pre-eclampsia or eclampsia.
- The death rate from eclampsia in the UK is about 2%.
- Pre-eclampsia is the commonest cause of iatrogenic prematurity.
- Hypertension accounts for 12–25% of all antenatal admissions.
- Antenatal care, especially in the second half of pregnancy, is largely geared toward the detection of hypertension and pre-eclampsia.

Clinical features

Hypertension in pregnancy may be divided into pre-existing hypertension, pregnancy-induced hypertension and pre-eclampsia. There are several definitions of 'hypertension' and these are discussed on p. 11.

Pre-existing hypertension

- Some women may have been diagnosed as hypertensive prior to pregnancy.
- If hypertension is noted for the first time in the first trimester, it is likely that it is a chronic, pre-existing problem, since pregnancy-induced hypertension (including pre-eclampsia) usually, but not invariably, appears in the second half of pregnancy.
- Diagnosis of pre-existing hypertension may, on occasion, only be made retrospectively, i.e. after delivery when the blood pressure has not returned to normal.
- Hypertension in any young person should not be attributed to essential (idiopathic) hypertension before secondary causes such as renal or cardiac disease, and rarely Cushing's syndrome, Conn's syndrome or phaeochromocytoma have been excluded.

- Women presenting with hypertension for the first time in early pregnancy should be examined for clues to a possible secondary cause. This should include examination of the femoral pulses (looking for radiofemoral delay suggesting coarctation of the aorta) and a search for renal bruits (possible renal artery stenosis).

- A simple screen with serum creatinine, urea (to exclude renal impairment), and electrolytes (to exclude hypokalaemia, which may suggest Conn's syndrome) should be performed. Urinary catecholamines should be measured in cases suggestive of phaeochromocytoma (see chapter 7).

- Women with pre-existing hypertension from whatever cause are at increased risk of superimposed pre-eclampsia, small for gestational age (SGA) infants, and placental abruption. Consequently, the perinatal mortality and premature delivery rates are increased in this population.

- If a woman is sufficiently hypertensive to require treatment before pregnancy, the risk of pre-eclampsia in pregnancy is approximately doubled. For those with severe hypertension (diastolic blood pressure >110 before 20 weeks' gestation), the risk of pre-eclampsia in one study was over 46%. These women are also at particular risk of early-onset pre-eclampsia.

Pregnancy-induced hypertension

- Pregnancy-induced hypertension and pre-eclampsia usually appear in the second half of pregnancy and resolve within 6 weeks of delivery, although blood pressure may remain elevated up to 3 months postpartum.

- Pregnancy-induced hypertension may be defined as hypertension occurring in the second half of pregnancy but in the absence of proteinuria or any other features of pre-eclampsia (Table 1.1). The distinction between pregnancy-induced hypertension and pre-eclampsia may be difficult, especially as many of the definitions of pre-eclampsia are based solely on hypertension.

- Differentiation between pre-existing and pregnancy-induced hypertension is not important when considering if, how and when to institute treatment, because the drugs suitable for the treatment of hypertension in pregnancy are the same for both conditions (Table 1.2).

- The distinction between pre-eclampsia and pregnancy-induced hypertension is however important since pre-eclampsia is associated with a worse pregnancy outcome.

- If hypertension develops after 20 weeks, the likelihood of progression to pre-eclampsia is about 15%. This risk is related to the gestation at presentation of pregnancy-induced hypertension. Thus for hypertension presenting before 30 weeks, the risk is about 40%, but if it presents after 38 weeks, the risk is only 7%.

- Pregnancy-induced hypertension tends to recur in subsequent pregnancies. Some women remain hypertensive following a pregnancy complicated by

Table 1.1 – Clinical features of pre-eclampsia

Symptoms
Headache/flashing lights
Epigastric/right upper quadrant pain
Nausea/vomiting
Rapidly increasing/severe swelling of face, fingers or legs
Signs
Pregnancy-induced hypertension (see p. 5)
Proteinuria (new onset)
Rapidly progressive oedema
Convulsions, mental disorientation
Intrauterine growth restriction/intrauterine death
Placental abruption
Investigations (Interpret with reference to normal values in pregnancy, Appendix 2 and inside back cover)
24-hour urinary protein excretion >0.3 g
Raised serum uric acid level
Thrombocytopenia
Prolonged clotting times
Raised serum creatinine and urea levels
Increased haematocrit and haemoglobin levels
Abnormal liver function tests, particularly raised transaminases
Reduced fetal growth, oligohydramnios
Abnormal uterine artery Doppler (bilateral notches at 24 weeks predict pre-eclampsia)
Abnormal umbilical artery Doppler (shows fetal compromise)

Table 1.2 – Drugs used to treat hypertension in pregnancy

Drug	Indication	Starting dose	Maximum dose	Contraindications	Safe when breast-feeding?
Methyldopa	First-line therapy	250 mg b.d.	1 g t.d.s.	Depression	Yes
Nifedipine	Second-line therapy	10 mg slow-release b.d.	40 mg slow-release b.d.		Yes
Hydralazine	Second-line therapy	25 mg t.d.s.	75 mg q.d.s.		Yes
Labetalol*	Third-line therapy	100 mg b.d.	500 mg t.d.s.	Asthma	Yes
α-blockers e.g. doxazocin	Third-line therapy	1 mg o.d.	8 mg o.d.		Yes†

*May be used as first-line therapy in the third trimester. †Doxazocin accumulates in breastmilk; prazocin should be used instead.

pregnancy-induced hypertension. Women with pregnancy-induced hypertension have an increased risk of hypertension in later life.

Pre-eclampsia

- Pre-eclampsia is a pregnancy-specific multi-system disorder of protean manifestation.
- Women with pre-eclampsia are usually asymptomatic when the disease is first manifest.
- Diffuse vascular endothelial dysfunction may cause widespread circulatory disturbances, involving the renal, hepatic, cardiovascular, central nervous and coagulation systems.
- Although hypertension and proteinuria are the most common manifestations of pre-eclampsia, they may be late or mild features, and the wider spectrum of the disorder should always be considered.
- Women may present with headache, visual disturbance, epigastric or right upper quadrant pain, nausea, vomiting or rapidly progressive oedema.
- The 'classic' signs are hypertension, proteinuria and oedema, but their absence does not exclude the diagnosis.
- The disorder is remarkably heterogeneous, with enormous variation in the severity, timing, progression and order of onset of different clinical features.

- Manifestations of pre-eclampsia (including eclampsia) may present ante-, intrapartum or postpartum.
- Effects on the kidney result in decreased glomerular filtration rate (GFR), proteinuria, a rise in serum creatinine and/or serum uric acid levels and oliguria.
- Hyperuricaemia also results from placental ischaemia accelerating trophoblast turnover and the production of purines (substrate for xanthine oxidase).
- Other features of the syndrome include a reduced plasma volume, haemoconcentration, abnormal liver function and thrombocytopenia.
- HELLP syndrome (one variant of pre-eclampsia) includes **H**aemolysis, **E**levated **L**iver enzymes and **L**ow **P**latelets, and may be associated with severe disseminated intravascular coagulation (DIC) (see chapter 11, p. 212).
- Several possible crises (Table 1.3) may develop.
- The commonest causes of death in pre-eclampsia are cerebral haemorrhage and adult respiratory distress syndrome.
- The placental manifestations lead to intrauterine growth restriction (IUGR), placental abruption and, in severe cases, intrauterine death.

Eclampsia

- Eclampsia may be defined as a tonic clonic (grand mal) convulsion occurring in association with features of pre-eclampsia (although the diagnosis may only be possible in retrospect) (Table 1.1).
- More than one-third of women experience their first convulsion before the development of hypertension and proteinuria.

Table 1.3 – Crises in pre-eclampsia

Eclampsia
HELLP syndrome
Pulmonary oedema
Placental abruption
Cerebral haemorrhage
Disseminated intravascular coagulation
Renal failure
Hepatic rupture

- Three-quarters of women with eclampsia in the UK have their first convulsion in hospital.

- Convulsions may occur antepartum (38%), intrapartum (18%) or postpartum (44%).

- Teenagers are three times more likely to suffer eclampsia than older women.

- Although eclampsia, like pre-eclampsia, is more common in primiparous women, 18% of women with eclampsia are multiparous without a previous history of pre-eclampsia.

- Eclampsia may be associated with ischaemic stroke with cerebral vasospasm and oedema. Neurological deficits usually resolve.

- Cortical blindness (usually reversible) is a well-described, although rare association of pre-eclampsia/eclampsia.

Pathogenesis

- This involves a genetic predisposition. The risk of pre-eclampsia is increased eight-fold for the woman with a sister who has had pre-eclampsia and four-fold if the mother was affected.

- Pre-eclampsia and otherwise idiopathic IUGR are part of the same disease spectrum and both relate to a problem of placentation (occurring in the first half of pregnancy) and consequent placental ischaemia. They differ with regard to the extent of the maternal response (developing in the second half of pregnancy).

- Placentation and trophoblast invasion is abnormal. It is uteroplacental ischaemia, whether due to poor implantation in underlying microvascular disease, or under-perfusion of a relatively large placenta (e.g. in a pregnancy complicated by diabetes, a multiple pregnancy, or a hydropic fetus) that is the common feature in pre-eclamptic pregnancies.

- The pathophysiology of pre-eclampsia and IUGR involves a lack of vascular adaptation to pregnancy. The invading placenta is unable to optimise its blood supply from maternal uterine vessels. The spiral arteries fail to adapt to become high-capacitance, low-resistance vessels.

- The precise mechanism by which the ischaemic placenta leads to the widespread endothelial cell damage that characterises the maternal syndrome is not known. Theories include lipid peroxidation stimulated by oxygen free radicals (reactive oxygen species) and increased deportation of syncytiotrophoblast microvillous membranes (STMMs). Both lipid peroxides and STMMs are harmful to maternal endothelium.

- Endothelial cell activation leads to increased capillary permeability, increased endothelial expression of cell adhesion molecules and prothrombotic factors, platelet thrombosis and increased vascular tone.

- In pregnancies complicated by pre-eclampsia, there is a decrease in prostacyclin synthesis and an increase in thromboxane A_2 (TXA_2) synthesis. It is thought that this reversal in prostanoid balance contributes to the platelet activation and vasoconstriction.

■ There is some evidence for defective production or decreased bioavailability of nitric oxide, an endogenous vasodilator, in pre-eclampsia.

■ The vasoconstrictive and pro-aggregative properties of TXA_2 may contribute to the histological finding of atherosis and thrombotic lesions seen in the spiral arteries of the uteroplacental circulation.

Risk factors

The risk factors include genetic, obstetric and medical factors, each of which will be discussed in turn.

Genetic factors

■ Women whose mothers had pre-eclampsia, have a 20–25% risk of developing pre-eclampsia.

■ In women with a sister with a history of pre-eclampsia, the risk may be as high as 35–40%.

Obstetric factors

■ Primiparity
■ Multiple pregnancy
■ Previous pre-eclampsia
■ Hydrops with a large placenta
■ Hydatidiform mole
■ Triploidy (particular association with very early onset [before 24 weeks' gestation] pre-eclampsia).

Medical factors

■ Pre-existing hypertension
■ Renal disease (even without functional renal impairment)
■ Diabetes (pre-existing or gestational)
■ Antiphospholipid antibodies (see chapter 8)
■ Connective tissue disease (see chapter 8)
■ Inherited thrombophilia (see chapter 3). There is an association with early-onset pre-eclampsia in some populations.

Diagnosis

- Because women with pre-eclampsia may be asymptomatic, much antenatal care is directed towards screening for this condition.
- In the first instance, this is done by measuring the blood pressure and checking the urine for protein.
- There is no diagnostic test for pre-eclampsia, but there are 'pointers' to the diagnosis (Table 1.1).
- There are several different definitions for hypertension in pregnancy, but most are based on a diastolic blood pressure >90 mmHg on two occasions or a diastolic blood pressure of >110 mmHg on a single occasion.
- Since it is the rise in blood pressure that may be important, rather than the absolute value, some definitions include a systolic blood pressure of 30 mmHg above the earliest recorded pregnancy reading or a diastolic increase of 15–25 mmHg.
- Proteinuric pre-eclampsia is defined as hypertension together with >0.3 g/24 hours proteinuria. 'Dipstick proteinuria', which is very inaccurate, must always be confirmed with a 24-hour urinary collection.
- These definitions of pre-eclampsia are very simplistic, since pre-eclampsia is a syndrome that may affect any system in the mother and indeed the fetus. In practice, the diagnosis is made when there is a constellation of recognised features (Table 1.1).
- It is the association of hypertension with these features that allows distinction of pre-eclampsia from pre-existing hypertension without superimposed pre-eclampsia and pregnancy-induced hypertension.

Management

Management of women with hypertension in pregnancy can be considered as:

- Screening for pre-eclampsia (regular blood tests, urinalysis)
- Treatment of hypertension
- Fetal surveillance
- Decision regarding timing of delivery.

Mild cases, especially where there is no evidence of pre-eclampsia, may be managed as outpatients.

If there is new onset hypertension and proteinuria, the woman should be admitted for assessment and will usually need to remain in hospital if pre-eclampsia is confirmed.

Monitoring for pre-eclampsia

- Regular checks of serum urea and creatinine, uric acid, haemoglobin, platelet count (and if thrombocytopenia is present and platelet count $<100 \times 10^9/l$, a coagulation screen) and liver function.

▪ Regular urinalysis, and if proteinuria ($\geq$1+) is detected, measurement of 24-hour protein excretion.

▪ Uterine artery Doppler blood flow examination at 20–24 weeks' gestation, looking particularly for the presence of a prediastolic 'notch'. A persistent high-resistance waveform is predictive of subsequent pre-eclampsia, IUGR and placental abruption. The negative predictive value is high and such screening is useful in high-risk women, for example, those with antiphospholipid syndrome or previous severe pre-eclampsia.

Treatment of hypertension

▪ Hypertension should be treated in its own right regardless of the assumed underlying pathology (pre-eclampsia, pre-existing hypertension, pregnancy-induced hypertension). This is because above a mean arterial (blood) pressure (MAP) of 150, there is loss of cerebral autoregulation and the mother is at risk of cerebral haemorrhage.

▪ MAP = D + 1/3 (S-D), where D = diastolic blood pressure and S = systolic blood pressure.

▪ The exact level of systolic or diastolic pressure at which to institute antihypertensive treatment is controversial depending on whether treatment is thought to be of benefit to fetal outcome; most physicians will treat at levels >140–170 mmHg systolic and >90–110 mmHg diastolic blood pressure. Treatment is mandatory if the blood pressure is $\geq$170/110.

▪ The target blood pressure is disputed; overzealous control runs the risk of jeopardising the uteroplacental circulation, but MAP should be maintained at <125 mmHg, e.g. 150/100.

▪ Treatment of pre-existing hypertension in pregnancy reduces the risk of severe hypertension (and therefore such severe complications as maternal cerebral haemorrhage) but there is no conclusive evidence to suggest that good control of blood pressure decreases the risk of superimposed proteinuric pre-eclampsia.

▪ Early in gestation, treatment of severe hypertension associated with pre-eclampsia that would otherwise be an indication for delivery, may allow prolongation of pregnancy (and therefore indirectly improve fetal outcome), but this does not actually modify the disease process.

▪ Later in pregnancy, treatment of hypertension may mask one of the important signs of pre-eclampsia. By treating the hypertension, clinicians are not treating but only palliating pre-eclampsia.

▪ Good control of blood pressure is important, but it should not preclude the definitive treatment of delivery if this is indicated for maternal (e.g. in HELLP syndrome) or fetal (e.g. with severe growth restriction) reasons.

Fetal surveillance

■ Women with either pre-existing hypertension or pre-eclampsia are at risk of IUGR, and management should therefore include regular ultrasound examination of the fetus to assess growth, liquor volume and umbilical artery blood flow.

■ Women developing pre-eclampsia who are likely to need delivery before 34 weeks' gestation should receive dexamethasone or betamethasone in order to induce fetal lung maturation. However, there is accumulating evidence that repeated antenatal steroid injections might be harmful to fetal growth and lung and neurodevelopment.

Decision regarding timing of delivery

■ The only cure for pre-eclampsia is delivery.

■ This should not be attempted before adequate control of blood pressure, coagulopathy, eclamptic seizures and haemodynamic stability is achieved.

■ In order to avoid neonatal deaths or long-term complications from prematurity, it is customary to try and prolong the pregnancy with 'expectant' management. This is often not possible for more than a few weeks, and in severe cases, only hours or days may be gained.

■ Indications for delivery are shown in Table 1.4. These are not necessarily absolute and obviously depend upon the gestational age and the speed of deterioration.

Drug treatment

Drugs used to treat hypertension in pregnancy (Table 1.2)

Table 1.4 – Indications for delivery

Inability to control blood pressure, e.g. maximal dose of three antihypertensive drugs
Rapidly worsening maternal biochemistry/haematology, e.g. falling platelet levels ($<100 \times 10^9$/l), coagulopathy, deteriorating liver or renal function, falling albumin levels (<20 g/l)
Eclampsia
Fetal distress/severe IUGR/reversed umbilical artery diastolic flow
Maternal symptoms, e.g. severe headache, epigastric pain

Methyldopa

Methyldopa is the drug of choice in pregnancy since it has been used for many years without any reports of serious adverse effects on the fetus or on children up to the age of 7 years. Methyldopa does have side effects, including depression, sedation and postural hypotension. Patients become tolerant to the sedative effect and this is less of a problem beyond 1 week after starting or increasing therapy. Depression or other side effects such as liver function test abnormalities, which persist or are severe, and haemolytic anaemia necessitate a change to a second-line drug.

β-blockers

β-blockers have fewer maternal side effects than methyldopa, but their safety in the fetus is not so well established. There is concern that these drugs may inhibit fetal growth when used long term (and started in the first trimester) throughout pregnancy, but claims of neonatal hypotension and hypoglycaemia have not been substantiated in the randomised, controlled trials performed. There is no evidence for the superiority of any one β-blocker over the others. β-blockers should not be given to women with a history of asthma. Guidelines of the International Society for the Study of Hypertension in Pregnancy (ISSHP) do not recommend the use of oral β-blockers for treatment of mild hypertension in pregnancy.

Some units still prefer labetalol, a combined α- and β-adrenergic blocker, to treat hypertension in pregnancy. However, because of the reservations outlined above concerning β-blockers, labetalol should be reserved for use in the third trimester, in combination with other drugs, or in women who are intolerant of first- or second-line agents. Parenteral labetalol has an important role in the intrapartum management of acute severe hypertension (see later).

Second-line drugs

Second-line drugs used for the treatment of hypertension in pregnancy include calcium antagonists (e.g. slow-release nifedipine) and oral hydralazine. These should be used in conjunction with methyldopa in women who fail to respond to monotherapy, or to replace methyldopa in the minority of women who are unable to tolerate it. Side effects include headache, facial flushing and oedema, and may necessitate withdrawal in some patients. α-adrenergic blockers are also safe and can be used as second- or third-line therapy.

Diuretics

Diuretics should only be used in pregnancy for the treatment of heart failure and pulmonary oedema. They are particularly hazardous and relatively contraindicated in pre-eclampsia because they cause further depletion of a reduced intravascular volume.

Angiotensin-converting enzyme inhibitors

The angiotensin-converting enzyme (ACE) inhibitors (e.g. ramipril, enalapril) should not be used in pregnancy because they may cause oligohydramnios, renal failure and hypotension in the fetus. Their use has been associated with decreased skull ossification, hypocalvaria and renal tubular dysgenesis, and there is also a risk of intrauterine death. Any woman on maintenance therapy with an ACE inhibitor should discontinue this (and if necessary switch to methyldopa) when pregnancy is confirmed. The use of these drugs in the first trimester is not associated with structural malformations, so it is acceptable to cease treatment early in pregnancy and not necessarily preconception.

Angiotensin II receptor blockers

There are little data concerning these newer agents (e.g. losartan) in pregnancy, but they are similar to the ACE inhibitors and therefore should be avoided.

Treatment of acute severe hypertension

- A protocol for the management of severe pre-eclampsia including criteria for transfer to intensive care should be available and agreed by obstetricians, anaesthetists, paediatricians and physicians.

- Women with severe pre-eclampsia should be managed in a high-dependency unit environment (on the labour ward if undelivered).

- Strict control of hypertension is the single most important pharmacological manoeuvre.

- Automated oscillometric devices may underestimate blood pressure compared to mercury sphygmomanometers.

- Many pre-eclamptic women have a reduced intravascular volume and all require pre-treatment with colloid before parenteral hypotensive therapy is started.

- Volume expansion optimises cardiac pre-load and improves renal and utero-placental blood flow. However, in the absence of blood loss, no patient should receive >500 ml of colloid without knowledge of the central venous pressure.

- The choice of antihypertensive agent for acute control varies but is usually hydralazine (intermittent i.v. bolus), labetalol (continuous i.v. infusion) or nifedipine (orally). Sublingual nifedipine causes too rapid a fall in blood pressure and uteroplacental perfusion and therefore should not be used.

- Vasodilators (hydralazine and nifedipine) cause headache and tachycardia in many patients, and are easier to use if the sympathetic nervous system is already inhibited with methyldopa.

- Nifedipine used in conjunction with magnesium sulphate may cause profound hypotension. In general, diuretic therapy should be avoided unless there is volume overload or pulmonary oedema.

- Continuous fetal heart rate monitoring is necessary to diagnose fetal distress that may be precipitated by antihypertensive therapy.
- Renal function and fluid balance must be monitored carefully. There is usually oliguria and poor tolerance to volume loading. Continuous oxygen saturation (SaO_2) monitoring is vital as aspiration of gastric contents and pulmonary oedema are always risks.
- Platelet count (and if low, clotting studies) and liver function should also be monitored.
- Management in the most critically ill patient must be based on haemodynamic monitoring with central venous pressure and intra-arterial lines.
- Right atrial pressure (especially if normal or high) may not always accurately reflect left atrial pressure and a pulmonary artery catheter may occasionally be indicated.

Management of eclampsia

- The drug of choice for primary and secondary prophylaxis in eclampsia is magnesium sulphate. This probably acts as a cerebral vasodilator.
- Eclampsia should be treated with i.v. magnesium sulphate followed by an infusion (for 24–48 hours after delivery or after the last seizure) to prevent further seizures.
- Seizure prophylaxis may be given to pre-eclamptics (especially those who have continued signs of cerebral irritation, such as agitation and clonus, despite good blood pressure control) as primary prophylaxis for eclampsia, but the case for routine prophylaxis in all cases of severe pre-eclampsia has not been proven.
- Magnesium sulphate is given as a loading dose of 4 g (diluted to 40 ml) over 5–10 minutes, followed by a maintenance infusion of 1 g/hour.
- Recurrent seizures should be treated by a further bolus of 2 g.
- Side effects of parenteral magnesium sulphate include neuromuscular blockade and loss of tendon reflexes, double vision and slurred speech, respiratory depression and cardiac arrest. Its use necessitates close monitoring of the respiratory rate, oxygen saturation, electrocardiogram, and tendon reflexes.
- If the woman is oliguric, has liver or renal impairment, or has a further convulsion, serum magnesium levels should be monitored (therapeutic range 2–4 mmol/l).

Management of delivery

- Women with pre-eclampsia are encouraged to have regional analgesia/anaesthesia in labour or for caesarean section.
- This helps control of hypertension by reduction of pre- and after-load and by

providing adequate analgesia. It also avoids the fluctuations in blood pressure associated with general anaesthesia and intubation.

- In the presence of thrombocytopenia, regional blockade may not be deemed safe, and general anaesthesia becomes necessary for caesarean section. Most obstetric anaesthetists use a cut-off for the platelet count of $60-70 \times 10^9/l$.

- Ergometrine should be avoided as it may produce an acute rise in blood pressure.

Postpartum management

- Although delivery removes the cause of pre-eclampsia, the manifestations, particularly hypertension, may take many weeks to resolve. There is often transient deterioration in the clinical state following delivery.

- Therefore, women require intensive monitoring following delivery with attention to blood pressure control, fluid balance, haematology and biochemistry.

- Diuresis usually occurs spontaneously, but is often preceded by a period of oliguria.

Oliguria

- Oliguria is a normal feature of pre-eclampsia, especially following operative delivery or after induction of labour with Syntocinon.

- The risk of pulmonary oedema from fluid overload continues postpartum and it is safer to err on the side of volume depletion and mild renal impairment than to treat immediate postpartum oliguria with aggressive volume replacement. This strategy is at variance with that used in other causes of oliguria presenting to intensive care units.

- If an infusion of Syntocinon is deemed necessary, this may be administered in a more concentrated form (e.g. through a syringe driver) to avoid excess fluid.

- Diuretics are usually inappropriate in the management of postpartum oliguria, unless there are obvious signs of fluid overload or pulmonary oedema.

- There is no demonstrable long-term benefit from the use of dopamine in this setting.

- The proteinuria also resolves spontaneously unless there is underlying renal pathology, but again may take several weeks or months to do so.

Hypertension

- Postpartum hypertension is common and often not anticipated. The blood pressure rises after normal pregnancy, often not reaching a peak until 3 or 4 days postpartum. Consequently, although normotensive immediately following delivery, women with hypertension during pregnancy may become hypertensive again within the first week postpartum. This is often apparent prior to planned discharge and may prolong the stay in hospital until the hypertension is brought under control.

■ Methyldopa should be avoided postpartum because of its tendency to cause depression.

■ β-blockers (e.g. atenolol 50–100 mg o.d.), with the addition of a calcium antagonist (e.g. slow-release nifedipine 10–20 mg b.d.) and/or an ACE inhibitor (e.g. enalapril 5–10 mg o.d.) if required, are appropriate for the treatment of postpartum hypertension.

■ In women who develop hypertension during pregnancy, it is usually possible to stop antihypertensive medication within 6 weeks postpartum.

■ All the drugs discussed earlier, including the ACE inhibitors, are safe to use in a woman who is breast-feeding.

■ For women with pre-existing hypertension, it is usual to switch from methyldopa to the patient's previous antihypertensive regime after delivery.

■ Diuretics are usually avoided in breast-feeding mothers because of the associated side effect of increased thirst.

Prophylaxis

Low-dose aspirin

■ The rationale for the use of low-dose aspirin is that it inhibits platelet cyclo-oxygenase and therefore TXA_2 synthesis.

■ Meta-analysis of all trials of antiplatelet therapy for the prophylaxis of pre-eclampsia shows a 15% reduction in the incidence of pre-eclampsia in women taking antiplatelet therapy. However 90 women need to be treated with low-dose aspirin to prevent one case of pre-eclampsia.

■ The results of individual large randomised trials such as the MRC Collaborative Low-dose Aspirin Study in Pregnancy (CLASP) trial suggest that aspirin may be effective in reducing the risk of early-onset pre-eclampsia (i.e. that necessitating delivery before 32 weeks' gestation).

■ Importantly, there is good evidence for the safety of low-dose aspirin use in pregnancy. It would therefore seem reasonable to prescribe prophylactic aspirin (75 mg/day) for women with the following conditions:
  – Hypertension and renal disease
  – Hypertension and diabetes
  – Women at high risk of pre-eclampsia and in particular early onset pre-eclampsia
  – Women who have had recurrent or severe pre-eclampsia in previous pregnancies.

- There is evidence that aspirin reduces the incidence of pre-eclampsia and other adverse pregnancy outcomes in women with acquired thrombophilia (antiphospholipid syndrome).
- If aspirin is used, therapy should commence at or before 12 weeks' gestation.

Calcium

Although meta-analyses have supported a lowering of the risk of pre-eclampsia with calcium supplementation in pregnancy, a large trial of over 4500 women found no difference in the incidence of pre-eclampsia between 2 g calcium and placebo.

Antioxidants

- The rationale for the use of antioxidants is that they are free radical scavengers. Free radicals and oxidative stress contribute to the pathogenesis of pre-eclampsia (see earlier).
- Supplementation with vitamin C 1000 mg/day and vitamin E 400 iu/day from 18–22 weeks' gestation in a high-risk population (previous history of pre-eclampsia or abnormal uterine artery Doppler scan) was associated with a greater than 50% reduction in the incidence of pre-eclampsia.
- Further multi-centre trials are in progress to confirm the beneficial effect in high-risk women and assess the effect in low-risk women.

Folic acid

- Hyperhomocysteinaemia and homozygosity for the thermolabile mutation of methylene tetrahydrofolate reductase (MTHFR) have been associated with early-onset pre-eclampsia in some populations.
- Homocysteine levels are reduced with folate supplementation.
- Supplementation with folic acid 5 mg/day is not harmful in pregnancy.
- Randomised studies are needed to determine any potential beneficial effect of folic acid in women with previous pre-eclampsia and the MTHFR mutation or hyperhomocysteinaemia.

Recurrence/pre-pregnancy counselling

- Women who have pre-eclampsia in their first pregnancy have about a 10% risk of developing pre-eclampsia in their second pregnancy.
- This risk is increased if they have an underlying medical risk factor such as pre-existing hypertension, renal disease or antiphospholipid syndrome, or if they had early onset pre-eclampsia or HELLP syndrome.

Hypertensive disorders in pregnancy – points to remember

- Hypertension is the commonest medical problem in pregnancy.
- Pre-eclampsia is the second commonest cause of maternal death in the UK.
- Pre-eclampsia is a heterogeneous multi-system endothelial disorder that causes more effects than just hypertension and proteinuria.
- Methyldopa is the drug of choice for treatment of hypertension in pregnancy.
- Eclampsia may pre-date hypertension and proteinuria.
- Women with pre-eclampsia require close monitoring, with particular regard to symptoms, blood pressure, renal and liver function, platelet count and fetal well-being.
- Delivery is the only cure for pre-eclampsia and this may be indicated for fetal or maternal reasons.
- Women with hypertension in pregnancy often require treatment with postpartum antihypertensives, but methyldopa should be avoided.
- Oliguria is a normal feature in the immediate postpartum period and should not be treated with large volumes of i.v. fluids, except if there is objective evidence of volume depletion.
- Normal maintenance antihypertensive therapy for women with pre-existing hypertension can replace methyldopa therapy after delivery, and these drugs are safe to use when breast-feeding.

Further reading

Chappell, L.C., Seed, P.T. and Briley, A.L. et al. (1999) Effect of antioxidants on the occurrence of pre-eclampsia in women at increased risk: a randomised trial. *Lancet* **354,** 810–816.

Department of Health, Welsh Office, Scottish Home and Health Department and Department of Health and Social Services, Northern Ireland (1998) *Confidential Enquiries into Maternal Deaths in the United Kingdom 1994–96.* London: HMSO.

Knight, M., Duley, L., Henderson-Smart, D.J. and King, J.F. (2000) Antiplatelet agents for preventing and treating pre-eclampsia (Cochrane Review). In: *The Cochrane Library,* Issue 3, Oxford: Update Software.

Magee, L.A., Ornstein, M.P. and von Dadelszen, P. (1999) Management of hypertension in pregnancy. *Br. Med. J.,* **318,** 1332–1336.

McCowan, L.M.E., Buist, R.G., North, R.A. and Gamble, G. (1996) Perinatal morbidity in chronic hypertension. *Br. J. Obstet. Gynaecol.,* **103,** 123–129.

Redman, C.W.G. and Roberts, J.M. (1993) Management of pre-eclampsia. *Lancet,* **341,** 1451–1454.

Saudan, P., Brown, M.A., Buddle, M.L. and Jones, M. (1998) Does gestational hypertension become pre-eclampsia. *Br. J. Obstet. Gynaecol.,* **105,** 1177–1184.

The Eclampsia Trial Collaborative Group (1995) Which anticonvulsant for women with eclampsia? Evidence from the Collaborative Eclampsia Trial. *Lancet,* **345,** 1455–1463.

Williams, D.J. and deSwiet, M. (1997) The pathophysiology of pre-eclampsia. *Intensive Care Med.,* **23,** 620–629.

CHAPTER 2

Heart disease

Cardiovascular adaptation to pregnancy

(Table 2.1)

- Physiological changes begin early in gestation and the primary event is probably peripheral vasodilatation. This is mediated by endothelium-dependent factors, including nitric oxide synthesis upregulated by oestradiol and possibly vasodilatory prostaglandins (PGI_2).

- Peripheral vasodilation leads to a fall in systemic vascular resistance and to compensate for this, the cardiac output increases by around 40% during pregnancy. This is achieved predominantly via an increase in stroke volume, but also by a lesser increase in heart rate.

- These changes begin early in pregnancy and by 8 weeks' gestation the cardiac output has already increased by 20%.

- The maximum cardiac output is found at about 20–28 weeks' gestation. There is a minimal fall at term. An increase in stroke volume is possible due to the early increase in ventricular wall muscle mass and end-diastolic volume (but not end-diastolic pressure) seen in pregnancy. The heart is physiologically dilated and myocardial contractility is increased.

- Although stroke volume declines towards term, the increase in maternal heart rate (10–20 b.p.m.) is maintained, thus preserving the increased cardiac output.

- There is a profound effect of maternal position towards term upon the haemodynamic profile of both the mother and fetus. In the supine position, pressure of the gravid uterus on the inferior vena cava causes a reduction in venous return to the heart and a consequent fall in stroke volume and cardiac output. Turning from the lateral to the supine position may result in a 25%

Table 2.1 – Cardiovascular adaptation to pregnancy

Physiological variable	Direction of change	Degree/timing of change
Cardiac output	↑	40%
Stroke volume	↑	
Heart rate	↑	10–20 b.p.m.
Blood pressure	↓	First and second trimesters
	→	Third trimester
Central venous pressure	→	
Pulmonary capillary wedge pressure (PCWP)	→	
Systemic vascular resistance (SVR) and pulmonary vascular resistance(PVR)	↓	25–30%
Serum colloid osmotic pressure	↓	10–15%

↑: increased; ↓: decreased; →: unchanged.

reduction in cardiac output. Pregnant women should therefore be nursed in the left or right lateral position wherever possible. If the woman has to be kept on her back, the pelvis should be rotated so that the uterus drops forward and cardiac output as well as uteroplacental blood flow are optimised.

■ Reduced cardiac output is associated with a reduction in uterine blood flow and therefore in placental perfusion; this can compromise the fetus.

■ Although both blood volume and stroke volume increase in pregnancy, pulmonary capillary wedge pressure and central venous pressure do not increase significantly.

■ Pulmonary vascular resistance (PVR), like systemic vascular resistance (SVR), decreases significantly in normal pregnancy.

■ Although there is no increase in pulmonary capillary wedge pressure (PCWP), serum colloid osmotic pressure is reduced. The colloid oncotic pressure/pulmonary capillary wedge pressure gradient is reduced by 28%, making pregnant women particularly susceptible to pulmonary oedema.

■ Pulmonary oedema will be precipitated if there is either an increase in cardiac pre-load (such as infusion of fluids), or increased pulmonary capillary permeability (such as in pre-eclampsia), or both.

Intrapartum and postpartum haemodynamic changes

■ Labour is associated with further increases in cardiac output (15% in the first stage and 50% in the second stage). Uterine contractions lead to auto-transfusion of 300–500 ml of blood back into the circulation and the sympathetic response to pain and anxiety further elevate heart rate and blood pressure. Cardiac output is increased more during contractions but also between contractions.

- Following delivery, there is an immediate rise in cardiac output due to the relief of inferior vena cava obstruction and contraction of the uterus that empties blood into the systemic circulation. Cardiac output increases by 60–80% followed by a rapid decline to pre-labour values within about 1 hour of delivery. Transfer of fluid from the extravascular space increases venous return and stroke volume further.
- Those women with cardiovascular compromise are therefore most at risk of pulmonary oedema during the second stage of labour and the immediate postpartum period.
- Cardiac output has nearly returned to normal (pre-pregnancy values) 2 weeks after delivery, although some pathological changes (e.g. hypertension in preeclampsia) may take much longer (see chapter 1).

Normal findings on examination of cardiovascular system in pregnancy

These may include:

- Bounding/collapsing pulse
- Ejection systolic murmur (present in over 90% of pregnant women. May be quite loud and audible all over the precordium)
- Third heart sound
- Relative sinus tachycardia
- Ectopics
- Peripheral oedema.

Normal findings on ECG in pregnancy

These are partly related to changes in the position of the heart and may include:

- Atrial and ventricular ectopics
- Q-wave (small) and inverted T-wave in lead III
- ST segment depression and T-wave inversion inferior and lateral leads
- QRS axis leftward shift.

General considerations

Ideally, pre-pregnancy counselling of women with heart disease will allow detailed assessment of cardiac status, and any potential risk to be explained before conception. But although most women with heart defects are aware of the diagnosis, many pregnancies are not planned, and increasingly, immigrant women who may never have had a medical check-up present with previously undiagnosed heart disease in pregnancy.

The heart has relatively less reserve than the lungs (see p. 80). Whatever the underlying cause of cardiac insufficiency, the ability to tolerate pregnancy is related to the following:

- Presence of cyanosis (arterial oxygen saturation, 80%)
- Presence of pulmonary hypertension
- Haemodynamic significance of any lesion
- Functional class (New York Heart Association, NYHA) (Table 2.2).

Other predictors of cardiac events in pregnant women with heart disease include:

- History of transient ischaemic attacks or arrhythmias
- History of heart failure
- Left heart obstruction
- Myocardial dysfunction.

Cyanosis alone may not be as important in predicting poor outcome as the association of cyanosis with pulmonary hypertension typically in Eisenmenger's syndrome, poor functional class, or both.

Poor pregnancy outcome is more likely if the woman has a poor functional status (NYHA class III or IV) regardless of the specific lesion. Conversely, those in function classes I or II are likely to do well in pregnancy. Each case must be assessed individually, but those that require special consideration (even if asymptomatic) are women with the following conditions:

- Mitral stenosis (risk of pulmonary oedema)
- Marfan's syndrome (risk of aortic dissection or rupture)
- Pulmonary hypertension.

Table 2.2 – NYHA functional classification

Class I	No breathlessness/uncompromised
Class II	Breathlessness on severe exertion/slightly compromised
Class III	Breathlessness on mild exertion/moderately compromised
Class IV	Breathlessness at rest/severely compromised

Detailed assessment by a cardiologist, obstetrician, and obstetric anaesthetist with an agreed and documented plan for delivery is crucial.

Pulmonary hypertension

(See also later under Eisenmenger's syndrome p. 29.) Women with pulmonary hypertension from whatever cause are at increased risk during pregnancy. The maternal mortality rate is 30–50%. Pulmonary hypertension in the pregnant woman may be due to the following:

- Lung disease, e.g. cystic fibrosis
- Primary pulmonary hypertension
- Pulmonary veno-occlusive disease
- Eisenmenger's syndrome (usually an atrial septal defect/ventricular septal defect with pulmonary hypertension and a reversed shunt, i.e. right to left).

Fixed pulmonary vascular resistance (in contrast to the normal fall in pregnancy) means that these women cannot increase pulmonary blood flow to match the increased cardiac output and they tolerate pregnancy poorly. Therefore, such women are usually offered sterilisation, or if they do become pregnant, a termination. Termination itself is associated with maternal mortality but this is less than that associated with such a pregnancy allowed to progress.

Congenital heart disease

The incidence of congenital heart disease in pregnancy is increasing as women with more severe defects, who underwent corrective surgery as children, are now able to have children themselves. The most common congenital heart diseases in pregnancy are patent ductus arteriosus (PDA), atrial septal defect (ASD) and ventricular septal defect (VSD). Together these account for about 60% of cases.

Simple acyanotic defects and uncomplicated left-to-right shunts pose little problem, and women with defects of minimal haemodynamic significance do well in pregnancy. The more common defects will be considered individually.

Patent ductus arteriosus

- Most cases encountered in pregnancy nowadays have undergone surgical correction in childhood.
- Corrected cases pose no problems in pregnancy and do not require antibiotic prophylaxis.
- Uncorrected cases usually do well, but are at risk of congestive cardiac failure.
- If the woman has pulmonary hypertension, she has Eisenmenger's syndrome (see later).

Atrial septal defect

- Usually well tolerated in pregnancy.
- Women may deteriorate and become hypotensive if there is an increase in the left-to-right shunt following blood loss at delivery. This causes a drop in left ventricular output and coronary blood flow.
- Supraventricular arrhythmias are uncommon before the age of 40, but may rarely complicate pregnancy.

Ventricular septal defect

- Usually well tolerated in pregnancy unless the woman has Eisenmenger's syndrome (see later).

Congenital aortic stenosis

- Unlikely to cause problems unless the gradient is severe (>100 mmHg in the non-pregnant state).
- The risks with moderate-to-severe disease are angina, hypertension, heart failure, and sudden death.
- Symptoms (e.g. angina, dyspnoea, pre-syncope, syncope) as well as hypertension may be controlled with β-blockers provided left ventricular function is good.
- The development of resting tachycardia may indicate a failing left ventricle, unable to maintain the increased stroke volume of pregnancy.
- Complications mainly arise in those with severe aortic stenosis because of a restricted capacity to increase cardiac output.
- Balloon valvotomy may allow temporary relief of severe stenosis and continuation of the pregnancy in severe cases.

Coarctation of the aorta

- If diagnosed, this is usually corrected prior to pregnancy.
- The risks with uncorrected coarctation are angina, hypertension and congestive heart failure. There is also an association with aortic rupture and aortic dissection. These latter risks may be minimised by strict control of the blood pressure and β-blockade to decrease cardiac contractility.

Marfan's syndrome

In pregnancy, this syndrome carries the risk of aortic dissection and aortic rupture.

Predictors for dissection and rupture include:

■ Pre-existing or progressive aortic root dilatation
■ Positive family history of dissection or aortic rupture.

Management

■ Pregnancy is contraindicated if the aortic root is >4–4.5 cm.
■ Patients at high risk should be offered aortic root replacement prior to pregnancy.
■ β-blockers have been shown to reduce the rate of aortic dilatation and the risk of complications in patients with Marfan's syndrome. They should be continued or started in pregnant patients with aortic dilatation or hypertension.
■ Regular echocardiograms should be carried out to assess aortic root diameter.

Marfan's syndrome is inherited as an autosomal dominant disorder. Those with cardiac lesions tend to have offspring with cardiac abnormalities. The other features of Marfan's syndrome are as follows:

■ Increased height
■ Arm span greater than height
■ Arachnodactyly
■ Joint laxity
■ Depressed sternum
■ Highly arched palate
■ Dislocation of the lens.

Cyanotic congenital heart disease

This carries significant risks for mother and fetus. Problems include:

■ Worsening cyanosis because of increased right-to-left shunting secondary to falling peripheral vascular resistance
■ Thromboembolic risk increased because of polycythaemia (secondary to hypoxaemia)
■ Increased risk of fetal loss (especially if oxygen saturation <80–85%)
■ Associated pulmonary hypertension.

Fallot's tetralogy

Those without pulmonary vascular disease, may negotiate pregnancy successfully. There are two main concerns:

■ Paradoxical embolism through the right-to-left shunt causing cerebrovascular accidents
■ Effects of cyanosis and maternal hypoxaemia on the fetus

- Intrauterine growth restriction
- Increased risk of miscarriage
- Increased risk of spontaneous and iatrogenic prematurity.

These risks can be minimised by use of the following:

- Subcutaneous heparin prophylaxis
- Elective admission for bed rest and oxygen therapy to maximise oxygen saturation.

Eisenmenger's syndrome

If women with Eisenmenger's syndrome (50% maternal mortality) refuse termination of pregnancy, they require the following treatment:

- Prophylactic heparin
- Elective admission for bed rest and oxygen therapy.

Opinion varies as to whether these patients should be delivered by elective caesarean section and whether epidural anaesthesia is safe to use or not. The dangers relate to increasing the right-to-left shunt, which may be minimised by ensuring adequate hydration. Most women with Eisenmenger's syndrome who die as a result of pregnancy, do so after delivery, and often despite intensive and appropriate care. Principles of management include:

- Management in an intensive care environment with intensivists, anaesthetists, cardiologists and obstetricians with expertise in the care of those with complicated heart disease
- Using supplemental oxygen to reduce pulmonary vascular resistance
- Avoiding hypovolaemia; maintaining pre-load
- Avoiding thromboembolism; using thromboprophylaxis
- Avoiding pulmonary artery catheters; monitoring oxygen saturation, CVP, blood pressure
- Avoiding systemic vasodilation (therefore using caution with epidurals and Syntocinon)
- Considering selective pulmonary vasodilators, e.g. inhaled nitric oxide, i.v. prostacyclin, particularly peripartum.

Detailed consideration of women with complicated congenital heart disease, who may have undergone palliative surgery, is beyond the scope of this handbook, but the following are important considerations:

- The risk of ventricular failure (particularly when the right ventricle is acting as the systemic pumping chamber)
- Any residual pulmonary hypertension.

Most cases of simple defects corrected in infancy pose no problem in pregnancy.

Genetic counselling

- The risk of the fetus having a congenital heart defect is higher if the mother rather than the father has congenital heart disease. Overall, the risk is about 2–5% (i.e. well over double the risk in the general population).
- The level of risk depends on the specific lesion and is higher for outflow tract lesions. If the fetus is affected, it tends to have the same lesion.
- In women with an ASD, the risk of an ASD in the fetus is about 5–10%; for aortic stenosis, the risk is highest (18–20%).
- Both Marfan's and hypertrophic cardiomyopathy (HOCM) (see later) have autosomal dominant inheritance.
- Women with congenital heart disease should be referred for a detailed fetal cardiac ultrasound.

If the congenital heart defect in the parent was thought to be due to acquired abnormalities in pregnancy, e.g. to congenital rubella infection, the risk to any offspring is probably not increased.

Acquired heart disease

- Worldwide the acquired heart disease most likely to affect women wishing to have children is rheumatic heart disease. This is caused by rheumatic fever, which damages one or more of the heart valves. It is usually contracted in childhood and is now very rare in the UK.
- Rheumatic heart disease may present for the first time in pregnancy, especially in immigrant women who have never been examined previously by a doctor.
- Mitral stenosis accounts for 90% of rheumatic heart disease in pregnancy.

Mitral stenosis

Particularly if undiagnosed, this may be dangerous in pregnancy.

Symptoms

- May be asymptomatic
- Dyspnoea
- Cough (productive pink, frothy sputum or haemoptysis).

Signs

- Mitral facies

- Tapping, undisplaced apex beat
- Usually in sinus rhythm, unless advanced disease
- Loud first heart sound (S_1), loud pulmonary second sound (P_2), opening snap
- Low-pitched, mid-diastolic rumble
- Signs of pulmonary oedema.

Effect of pregnancy on mitral stenosis

- Even if a woman is asymptomatic at the beginning of pregnancy, she can deteriorate rapidly and develop pulmonary oedema.
- This is usually precipitated by a rise in the resting heart rate.
- This may be as a result of intercurrent infection, exercise, or secondary to a failure to adequately increase stroke volume.
- Tachycardia is particularly dangerous in mitral stenosis since diastolic filling of the left ventricle (which is slowed in mitral stenosis) is further decreased and there is a consequent fall in stroke volume and a rise in left atrial pressure precipitating pulmonary oedema.
- Most women who develop complications do so in the late second or third trimester or peri-partum period.
- Poor prognostic features for development of pulmonary oedema include:
  - Severe mitral stenosis as assessed by valve area
  - Presence of moderate to severe symptoms prior to pregnancy.

Management

- Pulmonary oedema should be treated with diuretics.
- β-blockers should be used to slow the heart rate and allow time for left atrial emptying.
- Atrial fibrillation should be treated aggressively with digoxin and β-blockers.
- In expert hands balloon valvotomy and closed mitral valvotomy have very good results in pregnancy, but are only suitable for non-calcified valves with minimal regurgitation.
- Surgical valvotomy carries higher risks, with fetal mortality rates of 5–15% for closed valvotomy and 15–33% for open valvotomy.
- If women with severe mitral stenosis attend prior to pregnancy, they should be offered surgery (open/closed/balloon mitral valvotomy or valve replacement) before embarking upon pregnancy.

Regurgitant valve disease

- Systemic vasodilation and a fall in peripheral vascular resistance reduce afterload and therefore act to reduce regurgitation.

- Both mitral and aortic regurgitation are well tolerated in pregnancy, provided there is no significant left ventricular dysfunction.
- Women with heart failure can be safely treated with diuretics, digoxin and hydralazine and/or nitrates as vasodilators to 'off load' the left ventricle.

Cardiomyopathies

Hypertrophic cardiomyopathy (HOCM)

Of these, 70% are familial with autosomal dominant inheritance.

Clinical features

- Chest pain or syncope, caused by left ventricular outflow tract obstruction
- Double apical pulsation (palpable fourth heart sound)
- Ejection systolic murmur (left ventricular outflow obstruction)
- Pan-systolic murmur (mitral regurgitation)
- Arrhythmias
- Heart failure.

Some women may be asymptomatic, the diagnosis having been made because of screening following a diagnosis of HOCM in a first-degree relative or echocardiography to investigate a heart murmur detected in pregnancy.

Effect of pregnancy on HOCM

- Mostly well tolerated in pregnancy and the stroke volume is usually able to increase.
- β-blockers should be continued or started in pregnancy for those women with symptoms.
- Epidural anaesthesia/analgesia carries the risk of hypotension with consequent increased left ventricular outflow tract obstruction.
- Any hypovolaemia will have the same effect and should be rapidly and adequately corrected.

Peripartum cardiomyopathy

This rare condition is specific to pregnancy. It is defined as the development of heart failure in the absence of a known cause and without any heart disease prior to the last month of pregnancy. Onset is usually in the first month after delivery, but may occur in the last month of pregnancy and up to 5 months postpartum.

Risk factors include:

- Multiple pregnancy

- Pregnancy complicated by hypertension
- Multiparity
- Advanced maternal age
- Afro-Caribbean race.

Symptoms

- Dyspnoea
- Reduced exercise tolerance
- Palpitations
- Pulmonary and/or peripheral oedema
- Symptoms relating to peripheral or cerebral emboli.

Signs

- Tachycardia
- Pulmonary oedema
- Congestive cardiac failure
- Dysrhythmias
- Signs of pulmonary, cerebral and systemic embolisation
- Systemic embolism occurs in 24–40% of those affected by peri-partum cardio-myopathy, and ischaemic stroke in about 5%.

Aetiology

This is unknown, but in different series a variable proportion (up to 50–75%) of cases have histological evidence of myocarditis on endomyocardial biopsy.

Diagnosis

- This requires echocardiography. The diagnostic criteria are:
  - Left ventricular ejection fraction (LVEF) <45%
  - Fractional shortening <30%
  - Left ventricular end-diastolic pressure (LVEDP) >2.7 cm/m^2
- Often, echocardiography shows the heart is enlarged with global dilation of all four chambers and markedly reduced left ventricular function.

Management

- Elective delivery if antenatal.
- Thromboprophylaxis. Anticoagulants are mandatory if there is severely impaired left ventricular dysfunction, intracardiac thrombus or arrhythmias.

- Conventional treatment for heart failure including diuretics, vasodilators (hydralazine and/or nitrates), digoxin, inotropes and, after delivery, angiotensin-converting enzyme (ACE) inhibitors.
- Immunosuppressive therapy may be considered in cases with myocarditis documented by endomyocardial biopsy, that fail to improve within 2 weeks of initiation of standard heart failure therapy.
- Cardiac transplantation may be the only option in severe cases unresponsive to conventional and full supportive management.

Prognosis and recurrence

- Maternal mortality rate is reported to be 25–50%, but a more recent study documented a 95% 5-year survival. Most case fatalities occur close to presentation.
- About 50% of patients make a spontaneous and full recovery.
- Prognosis depends on normalisation of left ventricular size and function within 6 months after delivery. Mortality is increased in those with persistent left ventricular dysfunction.
- Women should be counselled against further pregnancy if left ventricular size or function does not return to normal, since there is a significant risk of recurrence. Therefore, puerperal cardiomyopathy should not be 'casually' diagnosed and should be supported by echocardiography at least.
- For those whose cardiomyopathy resolves, the recurrence risk is not known but appears to be lower (0–25%). However, the contractile reserve may be impaired, even if the left ventricle size and function are normal.
- Subsequent pregnancies require high-risk collaborative care.

Artificial heart valves

If valve replacement is necessary in women of child-bearing age, there are two main considerations:

- Mechanical heart valves require life-long anticoagulation.
- Grafted-tissue heart valves (from pigs or humans) have the advantage that anticoagulation is not usually required, but bioprostheses deteriorate with accelerated rapidity during pregnancy.

Management

- Because of the risk of valve thrombosis, women with metal prosthetic heart valves must continue full anticoagulation throughout pregnancy.
- The interests of the mother and fetus are in conflict. Continuation of warfarin affords the mother the lowest risk of thrombosis, whereas for the fetus, war-

farin is associated with an increased risk of teratogenesis, miscarriage, still-birth, and intracerebral bleeding (see chapter 3, p. 47).

- High-dose s.c. low-molecular-weight heparin (LMWH) is safe for the fetus but is associated with a higher risk of thrombosis for the pregnant woman.
- The choice of anticoagulation regimen will depend on:
  - Position of the prosthesis (valves in the mitral position are more likely to thrombose than those in the aortic)
  - Type of valve replacement (old-fashioned ball and cage valves, e.g. Starr–Edwards, or single-tilting disc, e.g. Bjork–Shiley, are more thrombo-genic than the newer bi-leaflet valves, e.g. St Jude)
  - Patient choice. Some women are unhappy to accept any additional risk to the fetus.
- All women should be counselled thoroughly prior to pregnancy regarding potential risks to herself and her fetus
- There are three broad anticoagulant regimens:
  - Warfarin throughout pregnancy (close monitoring; INR 2.5–3.5)
  - Heparin between 6 and 12 weeks' gestation followed by warfarin
  - Heparin throughout (high-dose s.c. LMWH or unfractionated heparin)
- All women should discontinue warfarin for 10 days to 2 weeks prior to delivery to allow clearance of warfarin by the fetus. While awaiting delivery, full antico-agulant doses of either s.c. heparin or LMWH or i.v. heparin should be used. Heparin does not cross the placenta and has a very short half-life.
- S.c. heparin should be discontinued for labour and delivery. The dose of i.v. heparin is reduced to prophylactic levels (about 1000 units/hour).
- Full anticoagulant doses of heparin should be resumed after delivery.
- Warfarin may be restarted 3–5 days following delivery.
- In the event of an urgent need to deliver a fully anticoagulated patient, war-farin may be reversed with fresh frozen plasma (FFP) and vitamin K, and heparin and LMWH with protamine sulphate.

Antibiotic prophylaxis

- Prophylaxis used to cover delivery is usually advocated for women with struc-tural heart defects. The exceptions are those with a repaired PDA, those with an isolated ostium secundum ASD and those with mitral valve prolapse without regurgitation.
- It is mandatory for women with artificial heart valves and those with a previous episode of endocarditis.
- The current recommendations are amoxycillin 1 g i.v. or i.m. plus gentamicin 120 mg i.v. or i.m. at the onset of labour or ruptured membranes.
- For women who are penicillin allergic, vancomycin 1 g i.v. or teicoplanin 400 mg i.v. can be used instead of amoxycillin.

Ischaemic heart disease

- Myocardial infarction is uncommon in women of child-bearing age, but is becoming more frequent as older women are becoming pregnant.
- The mortality rate from ischaemic heart disease in pregnancy is increasing. There were eight deaths reported in the UK from 1991–1993 and six reported in the 1994–1996 confidential enquiry. The worldwide maternal death rate from acute myocardial infarction is over 20%.

Pathogenesis

- Most cases occur in smokers.
- Other risk factors include:
  - Diabetes
  - Obesity
  - Family history of ischaemic heart disease
  - Hypertension
  - Hypercholesterolaemia
  - Multigravidas older than 33 years.
- Acute myocardial infarction occurs most commonly in the third trimester, peri-partum and postpartum.
- The anterior wall of the left ventricle and the territory of the left anterior descending coronary artery are the commonest sites involved.
- Atherosclerosis is only a feature in under half of cases; these tend to be those presenting antepartum and with risk factors.
- Other causes of myocardial infarction are relatively more common in pregnancy and include:
  - Coronary thrombosis without atheroma
  - Coronary artery dissection (rare, but it has a particular association with the peri-partum period)
  - Coronary artery aneurysm, spasm or embolism
  - Congenital coronary anomalies
  - Cocaine abuse.

Management

- Low-dose aspirin (75–150 mg/day) is safe for use in pregnancy and should be continued or commenced in pregnancy for primary and secondary prophylaxis or in the acute management of myocardial infarction.
- Simvastatin and other lipid-lowering drugs are normally discontinued in pregnancy since high doses have caused skeletal malformations in rats and discontinuation for the relatively short duration of pregnancy is unlikely to impact

on long-term therapy for hyperlipidaemia. However post-marketing surveillance has not identified any increase in adverse pregnancy outcomes.

■ Management for acute ischaemia and infarction is as for the non-pregnant woman, with heparin, β-blockers and nitrates.

■ Thrombolytic therapy has been used successfully but there is a significant risk of bleeding.

■ For those with previous myocardial infarction, poor prognostic features for future pregnancy include residual left ventricular dysfunction and the presence of continuing ischaemia.

Dissection of thoracic aorta

There has been a recent increase in the number of maternal deaths from ruptured aneurysm of the thoracic aorta and its branches. Even if the diagnosis is made, the mortality rate associated with this condition is high.

Clinical features

■ Aortic dissection should be considered in any pregnant patient presenting with acute severe chest pain.

■ There may be symptoms or signs from territory supplied by the coronary, carotid, subclavian, spinal or common iliac arteries, or aortic regurgitation.

Pathogenesis

Pregnancy predisposes to aortic dissection possibly due to haemodynamic shear stress. Other risk factors include:

■ Marfan's syndrome
■ Ehlers–Danlos syndrome
■ Coarctation of the aorta.

Diagnosis

■ Chest X-ray is mandatory and may show mediastinal widening, but a normal chest X-ray does not exclude the diagnosis.

■ Diagnosis may be confirmed with transoesophageal echocardiography (TOE), computerised tomography (CT) or magnetic resonance imaging (MRI).

Arrhythmias

■ Although sinus tachycardia may be a feature of normal pregnancy, it requires investigation to exclude hyperthyroidism, respiratory or cardiac pathology and hypovolaemia or sepsis (see Section B, Table 2).

- Palpitations and dizziness are common symptoms in pregnancy.
- Investigation should include electrocardiography. This will exclude pre-excitation from accessory pathways such as in Wolff–Parkinson–White syndrome.
- 24-hour Holter monitoring should be performed if the history suggests frequent and troublesome arrhythmias.
- Atrial and ventricular premature beats are common in pregnancy, but have no adverse effects on the mother or fetus and require no further investigation.
- Atrial flutter and fibrillation are rare and paroxysmal SVT is the commonest arrhythmia encountered in pregnancy. It usually pre-dates the pregnancy but may become more frequent in pregnancy.
- If an arrhythmia is diagnosed, thyroid status must be tested and an echocardiogram performed to exclude structural heart disease.

Antiarrhythmic drugs in pregnancy

- Treatment is only required for life-threatening arrhythmias or SVTs that are frequent, persistent or symptomatic.
- It is best to use a drug used frequently in pregnancy such as digoxin, verapamil, or β-blockers (e.g. propranolol, sotalol).
- Adenosine is safe to use to terminate SVTs.
- Amiodarone should be avoided.
- Flecainide is the drug of choice for tachyarrhythmias in the fetus. There is evidence for its safety when used in the second and third trimesters. Less information is available for first trimester use, but this may be justified if β-blockers or verapamil do not control arrhythmias, especially as these often worsen in pregnancy.

Further reading

Avila, W.S., Grinberg, M., Snitcowsky, R. et al. (1995) Maternal and fetal outcome in pregnant women with Eisenmenger's syndrome. *Eur. Heart J.*, **16**, 460–464.

McCaffrey, F.M. and Sherman, F.S. (1995) Pregnancy and congenital heart disease: The Magee Women's Hospital. *J. Matern. Fet. Med.*, **4**, 152–159.

Morley, C.A. and Lim, B.A. (1995) The risks of delay in diagnosis of breathlessness in pregnancy. *Br. Med. J.*, **311**, 1083–1084.

Oakley, C.M. (1997) Heart Disease in Pregnancy. London: BMJ Publishing Group.

Pearson, G.D., Veille, J.C., Rahimtoola, S. et al. (2000) Peripartum Cardiomyopathy. National Heart, Lung and Blood Institute and Office of Rare Diseases (NIH). Workshop Recommendations and Review. *JAMA*, **283**, 1183–1188.

Roth, A. and Elkayam, U. (1996) Acute myocardial infarction associated with pregnancy. *Ann. Intern. Med.*, **125**, 751–757.

Sadler, L., McCowan, L., White, H. et al. (2000) Pregnancy outcomes and cardiac complications in women with mechanical, bioprosthetic and homograft valves. *Br. J. Obstet. Gynaecol.*, **107**, 245–253.

CHAPTER 3

Thromboembolic disease

Physiological changes	Thrombophilia
Scope of the problem	Diagnosis
Clinical features	Management
Pathogenesis and risk factors	Prophylaxis
Cerebral vein thrombosis	

Physiological changes

■ Changes in the coagulation system during pregnancy produce a physiological hypercoagulable state (presumably to stop bleeding following delivery).

■ The concentrations of certain clotting factors, particularly VIII, IX and X are increased. Fibrinogen levels rise significantly by up to 50%.

■ Fibrinolytic activity is decreased.

■ Concentrations of endogenous anticoagulants such as antithrombin and protein S fall. Thus pregnancy alters the balance within the coagulation system in favour of clotting, predisposing the woman both pregnant and in the postpartum period to venous thrombosis.

■ This additional risk is present from the first trimester and for at least 6 weeks following delivery.

■ The *in vitro* tests of clotting remain normal in the absence of anticoagulants or a coagulopathy.

■ Venous stasis in the lower limbs is associated with venodilation and decreased flow that is more marked on the left. This is due to compression of the left iliac vein by the right iliac artery and the ovarian artery. The iliac artery only crosses the vein on the left.

Scope of the problem

■ Thrombosis and thromboembolism are the leading causes of maternal mortality in the UK, and the second most common causes of maternal mortality in the USA.

■ Pulmonary embolism (PE) in pregnancy and the puerperium kills 15 women each year in the UK, and accounts for one in three of all direct maternal deaths.

■ Thromboembolism has been a leading cause of maternal mortality in the UK since the Confidential Enquiries into Maternal Deaths began.

■ Pregnancy increases the risk of thromboembolism six-fold, and caesarean section further increases this risk approximately 10–20-fold. Emergency caesarean section is associated with a higher risk than elective caesarean section.

■ The incidence of non-fatal pulmonary embolism and deep vein thrombosis (DVT) in pregnancy is about 0.1% in developed countries.

■ The risk of DVT after caesarean section is around 1–2%.

■ DVT increases the risk of further DVT and venous insufficiency in later life (65% in legs with previous DVT versus 22% in unaffected legs).

Clinical features

Deep vein thrombosis

■ There is a significant preponderance of left-sided DVT compared to right-sided DVT in pregnancy (ratio left:right = 9:1; left-sided = 85% in pregnancy versus 55% in non-pregnancy).

■ Compared to the non-pregnant patient, iliofemoral thrombosis is more common than popliteofemoral (72% in pregnancy versus 9% in non-pregnancy).

■ The classical features of swelling, redness, pain and tenderness of the calf are unreliable in pregnancy and clinical assessment alone will be wrong in 30–50% of cases.

■ Leg oedema (which may often be asymmetrical) is common in pregnancy without DVT.

Pulmonary embolism

■ A high index of suspicion is needed.

■ Breathlessness and pleuritic pain, particularly of sudden onset, should always be investigated.

■ Other features include cough and haemoptysis.

■ Large PEs may present with central chest pain and/or collapse with shock.

■ Examination may reveal tachypnoea, tachycardia, raised jugular venous pressure, a loud second heart sound and a right ventricular heave. With pulmonary infarction, a pleural rub and fever may also be present.

Pathogenesis and risk factors

Factors contributing to the increased risk of thromboembolism in pregnancy and the puerperium include the following:

Physiological changes common to all pregnant women
(see earlier)

- Haemostatic factors creating a procoagulant state from early pregnancy
- Venous stasis
- Trauma to the pelvic veins at the time of delivery.

Additional risk factors

- Obesity (>80 kg)
- Increased maternal age (>35 years)
- Increased maternal parity (four or more)
- Operative delivery (particularly emergency caesarean section)
- Thrombophilia (see later)
- Previous thromboembolism
- Prolonged bed rest/immobility
- Pre-eclampsia
- Gross varicose veins
- Hyperemesis/dehydration
- Ovarian hyperstimulation syndrome (particular association with internal jugular venous thrombosis).

Thrombophilia

- Women with thrombophilia are at increased risk of recurrent thromboembolic events in pregnancy or the puerperium.
- Thrombophilia may be divided into inherited and acquired forms (Table 3.1).
- A history of recurrent, atypical (e.g. axillary vein) or unprovoked (not associated with combined oral contraceptive, pregnancy, trauma or surgery) thromboembolism should stimulate a search for thrombophilia.
- Similarly, a family history of thromboembolism is important, since it may point to a diagnosis of inherited thrombophilia.
- Deficiencies of the naturally occurring anticoagulants protein C, protein S, and antithrombin (AT) are rare but are associated with high recurrence risks for thrombosis. These are approximately 12–17% (protein S deficiency), 22–26% (protein C deficiency) and 32–51% (AT deficiency).

Table 3.1 – Inherited and acquired thrombophilia

Inherited	Acquired
Protein C deficiency	Lupus anticoagulant
	Anticardiolipin antibodies
Protein S deficiency	
AT deficiency	Note: Antiphospholipid syndrome = lupus anticoagulant and/or anticardiolipin antibodies + thrombosis and/or recurrent miscarriage and/or fetal loss and/or delivery at or before 34 weeks' gestation due to severe pre-eclampsia/IUGR
FVL	
Prothrombin (PT) gene mutation	

AT: antithrombin; FVL: factor V Leiden; IUGR: intrauterine growth restriction; PT: prothrombin.

- The more recently discovered factor V Leiden (FVL – a single missense mutation in the factor V gene and the cause of 90% of cases of activated protein C resistance [APCR]) is present in about 5% of the UK population. The *G20210A* mutation of the prothrombin gene leads to elevated levels of prothrombin and is present in about 2% of the population. These thrombophilias are associated with a lower risk of recurrent thrombosis.

- FVL is inherited as an autosomal dominant trait inflicting on those heterozygous for the defect a life-long 5–10-fold increased risk of thrombosis. This risk may not manifest clinically unless there is a precipitating factor such as pregnancy, surgery or use of an oestrogen-containing oral contraceptive. The risk is higher for homozygotes.

- The prevalence of the prothrombin gene *G20210A* and FVL mutations in healthy subjects is dependent on the ethnicity and country of origin of the population under investigation. Low prevalences are found in Asians and Africans.

- The risk of thrombosis in women with thrombophilia is much higher in those with a personal compared to those with only a family history of thrombosis.

- Women with the less severe thrombophilias (e.g. FVL, prothrombin gene mutation) who have not themselves experienced a thrombosis can probably safely be managed in pregnancy with low-dose aspirin (see later under Prophylaxis). Use of heparin to cover delivery and the immediate postpartum period is justified.

- Inherited thrombophilia may be a factor in thrombosis occurring in pregnancy and the puerperium in up to 50% of women.

- The risk of recurrent thrombosis in antiphospholipid syndrome (APS) may be as high as 70%, and some of these women will be on long-term warfarin treatment outside pregnancy (see chapter 8, p. 146).

- Women with a previous history of thromboembolism should be screened for thrombophilia in the first trimester or preconceptually.

- Increased age is an important risk factor; a 40-year-old woman has a risk 100-fold that of a 20-year-old woman. Age also interacts with thrombophilia.

Adverse pregnancy outcome

- Several studies have suggested an association between adverse pregnancy outcome (pre-eclampsia, intrauterine growth restriction [IUGR], placental abruption, late fetal demise, recurrent early miscarriage, intrauterine death and stillbirth) and inherited thrombophilias, including those listed in Table 3.1, and homozygosity for the thermolabile mutation of methylene tetrahydro-folate reductase (MTHFR) causing mild hyper-homocysteinaemia. Other studies do not support this association in all populations.

- A beneficial effect for aspirin and/or heparin in the treatment of adverse pregnancy outcome in APS has been demonstrated, (see p. 149). No similar data exist for the inherited thrombophilias.

- Universal screening of women with previous poor obstetric histories for inherited thrombophilias is inappropriate, until the likelihood of recurrent adverse outcome and the results of randomised intervention studies in such women with thrombophilia are known.

Diagnosis

Deep vein thrombosis

- An objective diagnosis is vital because of the major implications in pregnancy of the:
  - Need for prolonged therapy
  - Potential need for prophylaxis in subsequent pregnancies
  - Concern regarding the future use of oestrogen-containing contraceptives
  - Subsequent use of hormone replacement therapy (HRT).

- The gold standard remains venography, which if performed with abdominal shielding is associated with negligible radiation to the fetus (Table 3.2).

- More convenient, less invasive and widely available is Doppler ultrasound. This tool is accurate in its detection of thrombi above the calf and below the inguinal ligament. Clots confined to the calf veins do not usually embolise and give rise to PE. The advantage of Doppler is that it may be repeated to exclude

Table 3.2 – Estimated radiation to the fetus associated with investigations for thromboembolism

Investigation	Radiation (μGy)
Chest X-ray	<10
Limited venography	<500
Unilateral venography without abdominal shield	3140
Perfusion lung scan (technetium-99m)	60–120
Ventilation lung scan	
Xenon-133	40–190
Technetium-99m	10–350
Pulmonary angiography	
Brachial route	<500
Femoral route	2210–3740

Note: Maximum recommended exposure in pregnancy = 50 000 μGy (5 rad).

extension of calf vein thrombi above the knee. Three features of thrombi are detectable with Doppler ultrasound:
1. Direct imaging of the clot
2. Lack of compressibility of the vein
3. Absence of distal distension of the vein during a Valsalva manoeuvre.

■ Impedance plethysmography has been less fully evaluated in pregnancy, but is safe.

■ D-dimers, widely used outside pregnancy in algorithms for diagnosis of thrombosis, are not helpful in pregnancy since the false-positive rate is high.

Pulmonary embolism

■ The chest X-ray is often normal, but is an essential part of investigation to exclude other important causes of breathlessness, chest pain or hypoxia. In cases of PE, it may show the following:
  – Areas of translucency in underperfused lung
  – Atelectasis
  – Wedge-shaped infarction
  – Pleural effusion.

■ The ECG may also be normal except for a sinus tachycardia. In cases of large PE, there may be the following:
  – Right-axis deviation

- Right-bundle branch block
- Peaked P-waves in lead II due to right atrial dilation
- The classical S_1, Q_3, T_3 pattern is rarely seen.

■ There is usually a raised white cell count and a polymorphonuclear leukocytosis.

■ Arterial blood gases reveal hypoxaemia and hypocapnia.

■ A useful screening test is to measure the oxygen saturation (using a pulse oximeter) at rest and after exercise, looking for resting hypoxia or a fall (>3–4%) after exercise.

■ Diagnosis must be confirmed with a lung scan. If the chest X-ray is normal, a perfusion scan alone (technetium-99m) may demonstrate underperfused areas. If the chest X-ray is abnormal and the cause of the abnormality is uncertain, an additional ventilation scan (xenon-133) will allow detection of ventilation/perfusion mismatch in cases of PE. The total radiation to the fetus from a lung scan is minimal and well below the recommended total pregnancy maximal dose for radiation workers in the USA (Table 3.2).

■ Pulmonary angiography is usually reserved for severe cases where localisation of the embolus prior to surgical or medical embolectomy is required.

■ Spiral CT, although usually avoided in pregnancy, involves minimal radiation to the fetus.

Management

■ Initial treatment is as for the non-pregnant patient. If there is a high level of clinical suspicion, treatment doses of i.v. heparin or s.c. low-molecular-weight heparin (LMWH) should be commenced prior to confirmatory diagnostic tests.

■ Larger doses (than in the non-pregnant woman) of i.v. heparin (e.g. 40 000 units/24 hours) are required.

■ I.v. heparin is given in doses adequate to prolong the activated partial thromboplastin time (APTT) by 1.5–2.0 times control for at least 5 days.

■ The platelet count should be checked 5–7 days after commencing heparin therapy.

■ Longer courses may be required if clinical improvement is not evident, or if scans fail to show some resolution after 5–7 days.

■ High-dose s.c. LMWH is now standard management of deep venous thrombosis outside pregnancy, and experience in pregnancy is growing. Doses are based on weight (e.g. enoxaparin [Clexane®] 1 mg/kg b.d.) and peak anti-Xa levels (3 hours post-injection) of 0.4–1.0 u/ml are the aim.

■ In cases of life-threatening PE, thrombolysis, pulmonary artery catheter break up of clot, and embolectomy have been successfully used.

- The use of vena caval filters should be restricted to cases of recurrent PE in the presence of demonstrable iliofemoral thrombosis, despite adequate full anticoagulation.
- Following acute-phase management with i.v. heparin or high-dose LMWH, some form of thromboprophylaxis must be continued for the rest of the pregnancy and the puerperium.
- This is usually with s.c. LMWH heparin (enoxaparin [Clexane®]; dalteparin [Fragmin®]). The dose of LMWH may be safely decreased from treatment doses to prophylactic doses (see later) after 1–3 months' treatment. An alternative is 10 000 units unfractionated heparin b.d.
- Intra- and postpartum management is discussed later under 'Prophylaxis'.

Prophylaxis

The following are drugs used for thromboprophylaxis and their side effects.

Warfarin

- Warfarin crosses the placenta, is teratogenic and must therefore be avoided during the first trimester.
- The teratogenic risk of chondrodysplasia punctata, nasal hypoplasia, growth restriction, short proximal limbs and other abnormalities is about 5%. The period of risk is between the 6th and 12th week of gestation, so conception on warfarin therapy is not dangerous, provided the warfarin is replaced by heparin within 2 weeks of the first missed period.
- The risk of miscarriage and stillbirth is also increased.
- The association with microcephaly and neurological abnormalities when warfarin is used in the second trimester may be related to over-anticoagulation of the mother, and therefore the fetus.
- There is a significant risk of both maternal (retroplacental) and fetal (intracerebral) bleeding when used in the third trimester, and particularly after 36 weeks' gestation.
- The use of warfarin for obstetric thromboprophylaxis in the second and early third trimesters should only be under close supervision and following thorough discussion with the woman.
- The single undisputed indication for warfarin use in pregnancy is for thromboprophylaxis in women with metal prosthetic heart valve replacements (see chapter 2, p. 34), in whom the risk of thrombosis is high, and for whom thrombosis carries a high mortality rate. These women require full anticoagulation throughout pregnancy.

Heparin

■ S.c. heparin, which does not cross the placenta and therefore has no adverse effects on the fetus, is the most commonly used mode of thromboprophylaxis in pregnancy in the UK.

■ The risk of heparin-induced osteoporosis is particularly pertinent in obstetrics, firstly because heparin use may last for up to 10 months, and secondly because pregnancy and breast-feeding cause reversible bone demineralisation (see chapter 8). There have been several reports of vertebral collapse associated with heparin use in pregnancy.

■ The incidence of symptomatic osteoporosis associated with unfractionated heparin use in pregnancy may be as high as 2%, and it is this risk that must be balanced against the risk of recurrent thromboembolism. The risk with LMWH is lower (0.2%).

■ Heparin-induced osteopenia may be subclinical, and studies have shown that thromboprophylaxis with unfractionated heparin in pregnancy may cause a 5% reduction in bone density, equivalent to 2 years' postmenopausal bone loss. Fortunately, however, bone density improves once heparin therapy is discontinued.

■ Thrombocytopenia is another rare but potentially dangerous side effect of heparin. There are two forms of heparin-induced thrombocytopenia:
1. An immediate-onset non-idiosyncratic reaction that is of little clinical importance
2. A later (6–10 days) idiosyncratic immune-mediated form that is more serious and associated with paradoxical thrombosis.

■ There are reports of heparin-induced thrombocytopenia in pregnancy, but in the UK this complication of heparin therapy is very unusual.

Low-molecular-weight heparins

■ LMWHs, produced by enzymatic or chemical breakdown of the heparin molecule, offer advantages over standard unfractionated heparins (UHs).

■ The most obvious advantage in obstetrics, where the timescale of prophylaxis is much longer than in surgery, is the increased bioavailability and longer half-life that together allow for once daily administration.

■ Because LMWHs are composed of shorter molecules than UHs, the ratio of anti-Xa (antithrombotic) to anti-IIa activity (anticoagulant), which is inversely proportional to the molecular weight, is increased. This property has led to claims of an improved clinical benefit (antithrombosis) to risk (inadvertent anticoagulation and bleeding) ratio.

■ LMWHs have less effect on platelet aggregation and less inhibition of platelet function than UH, and this reduces the risk of early thrombocytopenia. LMWHs are less capable than UH of activating resting platelets to release platelet factor IV, and they bind less well to platelet factor IV, thereby decreasing the risk of late-onset immune thrombocytopenia.

- LMWHs have been studied extensively outside pregnancy. They are certainly as effective and may well be safer than UH. Their use in pregnancy is now widespread because of their convenience and acceptability.

- LMWHs are associated with a lower risk of osteoporosis. Routine bone densitometry is not therefore indicated following use of prophylactic doses of LMWH throughout pregnancy.

- Some women develop a local allergic reaction to LMWH. If this occurs women usually develop a similar localised pruritic urticarial skin eruption to all forms of UH and LMWH. In these unusual cases, heparinoids such as Organon have been used successfully.

Prophylactic doses of heparin

- The increased circulating blood volume in pregnancy necessitates a higher dose of heparin (10 000 units b.d.) and LMWH (enoxaparin [Clexane®] 40 mg o.d.; dalteparin [Fragmin®] 5000 units o.d.), than is recommended outside pregnancy.

- During labour, or for women starting prophylaxis in labour, the dose of unfractionated heparin is reduced to 7500 units b.d.

- Heparin is usually given as self-administered, s.c. injections.

Aspirin

- Antiplatelet therapy has been shown to be effective in reducing the risk of venous thrombosis in surgical and medical patients. A recent study suggested the use of low-dose aspirin reduced the risk of thrombosis after orthopaedic surgery by 36%, even in some patients taking concomitant heparin prophylaxis.

- The use of aspirin as thromboprophylaxis in pregnancy has never been submitted to randomised, controlled trial but it is known that low-dose aspirin is safe in pregnancy.

- It does not seem unreasonable, therefore, to use aspirin in situations where the risk of thrombosis is not deemed high enough to warrant s.c. heparin use.

Indications for thromboprophylaxis

Since thromboprophylaxis with heparin or warfarin is not without the risks described earlier, a policy of universal thromboprophylaxis is not appropriate, and some assessment of individual risk is needed before deciding whether, and for how long, thromboprophylaxis is needed (Table 3.3). Such protocols differ between different obstetric units. When assessing the need for thromboprophylaxis in pregnancy, an accurate history of previous thromboembolic events is vital, and one should enquire whether a diagnosis of previous thromboembolism was objectively confirmed.

Table 3.3 – Protocol for obstetric thromboprophylaxis

Risk category	Risk factors	Prophylaxis
High risk	Previous thromboembolism + inherited thrombophilia	Antenatal s.c. heparin or LMWH
	Previous thromboembolism + antiphospholipid antibodies	*and* Intrapartum s.c. heparin or LMWH
	Previous thromboembolism + family history of thromboembolism	*and* Postpartum s.c. heparin or LMWH
	Recurrent thromboembolism	for 5 days followed by s.c. heparin or LMWH or warfarin
	AT deficiency even without previous thrombosis	for a total of 6 weeks
	Thromboembolism in current pregnancy	
Low risk	One previous thromboembolic episode (without a detectable thrombophilia or family history of thromboembolism)	Antenatal low-dose (75 mg) aspirin
		and Intrapartum s.c. heparin or LMWH
	Thrombophilia without a previous history of thrombosis (e.g. PS, PC deficiencies FVL, PT, aCL, LA)	*and* Postpartum as above for 6 weeks
Additional risk	≥3 points on risk assessment profile for delivery (see later)	Intrapartum subcutaneous heparin or LMWH *and* Postpartum s.c. heparin or LMWH for 3–5 days

FVL: factor V Leiden; PC: protein C; PS: protein S; PT: prothrombin gene mutation; aCL: anticardiolipin antibodies; LA: lupus anticoagulant.

High risk

- Antenatal, intrapartum and postpartum heparin prophylaxis is necessary for women who have had a previous thromboembolic event and who have a thrombophilia (hence the importance of screening all women with previous episodes of thrombosis). It is also required for women with a family history of thromboembolism, with thromboembolism in the current pregnancy, and with a history of more than one previous thromboembolic event.
- Women with AT deficiency, even if there is no past history of thrombosis, require heparin prophylaxis throughout pregnancy and the puerperium because of the high risk of thrombosis (see earlier).
- Women with antiphospholipid antibodies (lupus anticoagulant or anticardiolipin antibodies) should receive low-dose aspirin antenatally for fetal reasons (see chapter 8). If they have had a previous thromboembolic event, additional heparin throughout pregnancy is mandatory. Many of these women will have been receiving maintenance doses of warfarin outside pregnancy.

Low risk

- Women with a single previous thromboembolic event, but without a thrombophilia or a family history, especially if there was a clearly identifiable provoking factor for the thrombosis, do not require antenatal heparin. They should however receive heparin prophylaxis in labour and the puerperium, and may benefit from low-dose (75 mg/day) aspirin antenatally.
- Women diagnosed as having a thrombophilia (FVL, prothrombin gene mutation, protein S or C deficiency) via family studies, but who themselves have no personal history of thrombosis, may be managed according to the same protocol. Such cases need constant review since, if for example a woman with a known thrombophilia was admitted for pre-eclampsia or bed rest, this would be an indication to 'step up' the prophylaxis to heparin.
- Similarly, women with antiphospholipid syndrome but without previous thrombosis or fetal indications for heparin are managed with antenatal low-dose aspirin but should receive postpartum heparin for 5 days.

Additional risk factors

- The Royal College of Obstetricians and Gynaecologists (RCOG) has published recommendations for prophylaxis in obstetrics. These include a risk assessment profile for thromboembolism in caesarean section (Table 3.4). The RCOG recommendations do not stipulate which form of prophylaxis (i.e. s.c. heparin or leg stockings or intermittent pneumatic calf compression) should be used in women classified as 'moderate risk', i.e. those with only one or two risk factors. Interpretation of these recommendations is therefore variable,

Table 3.4 – Risk assessment profile for thromboembolism in caesarean section
(adapted, with permission, from RCOG)

Risk category	Clinical features	Suggested prophylactic measures
Low risk	Elective LSCS	Early mobilisation and hydration
	Uncomplicated pregnancy	
	No other risk factors	
Moderate risk	Emergency caesarean section in labour	S.c. heparin or mechanical methods
	Age >35 years	
	Obesity (>80 kg)	
	Para four or more	
	Gross varicose veins	
	Current infection	
	Pre-eclampsia	
	Immobility for >4 days prior to surgery	
	Major current illness, e.g. heart or lung disease, cancer, inflammatory bowel disease, nephrotic syndrome	
High risk	A patient with three or more moderate risk factors from list above	Heparin prophylaxis ± leg stockings
	Extended major pelvic or abdominal surgery, e.g. caesarean hysterectomy	
	Patients with a personal or family history of deep venous thrombosis, pulmonary embolism or thrombophilia; paralysis of lower limbs	
	Patients with antiphospholipid antibody	

Suggested doses of s.c. heparin are: 5000 units UH b.d. or 20 mg enoxaparin (Clexane®) o.d. or 2500 units dalteparin (Fragmin®) o.d. LSCS: lower segment caesarean section.

but some obstetric units would recommend heparin prophylaxis for all women undergoing emergency caesarean section in labour. Many units would also use a higher dose of heparin (e.g. enoxaparin [Clexane®] 40 mg o.d.; dalteparin [Fragmin®] 5000 units o.d.).

- Prophylaxis to cover delivery should not be limited to those undergoing caesarean section, since some women who die of pulmonary embolism following childbirth have had vaginal deliveries.
- Prophylaxis should be considered for obese, older women, and for those with other combinations of risk factors, even for vaginal delivery.
- An alternative risk assessment protocol for intrapartum prophylaxis is given in Table 3.5.

Table 3.5 – Alternative risk assessment profile for administration of intrapartum thromboprophylaxis (Calculate the total number of points for each patient depending on age, weight, mode of delivery and other risk factors, then refer to action plan.)

Points	Age	Weight	Delivery	Other
0	<35	<80 kg	Vaginal	
1	36–40	80–100 kg BMI >25	Elective caesarean section	– Para 4 or more – Gross varicose veins – Current infection – Pre-eclampsia – Immobility prior to surgery >4 days – Major current illness (e.g. heart or lung disease)
2	>40	100–120 kg BMI >30	Emergency caesarean section	Sickle-cell (SS or SC) disease
3		>120 kg BMI >35		– Extended major pelvic or abdominal surgery, e.g. caesarean hysterectomy – Personal history of DVT or PE – Thrombophilia – Paralysis of the lower limbs – Antiphospholipid antibody (aCL or LA)

Worked example: A 37-year-old woman weighing 72 kg and having an emergency caesarean section for pre-eclampsia would score 4 points (1 + 0 + 2 + 1).

Table 3.5 *continued* –
Prophylactic action plan depending on total number of risk points calculated from above

Total points (see example)	Action
0	Early mobilisation and hydration
1	Early mobilisation and hydration
2	TED stockings and consider heparin* + Early mobilisation and hydration
3 or more	heparin prophylaxis* + TED stockings, early mobilisation and hydration

*Heparin prophylaxis = Fragmin® 5000 units/day or Clexane® 40 mg/day (subcut) to start prior to delivery but after regional anaesthesia/analgesia or as soon as possible after delivery and continued for 5 days. TED: thromboembolic deterrent.

■ The time of greatest risk for thrombosis is around the time of delivery and the early puerperium. Therefore, women who qualify for intrapartum heparin prophylaxis alone can probably safely discontinue this after 3–5 days if they are fully mobile.

Antenatal management

■ Having decided into which risk category (Table 3.3) a women falls, she should be counselled appropriately. This is particularly so for 'high-risk' women regarding the relative risks of heparin-induced osteoporosis and recurrent thromboembolism.

Monitoring women receiving long-term heparin

■ A platelet count should be performed in all patients on heparin therapy to check for heparin-induced thrombocytopenia. Since immune/late heparin-induced thrombocytopenia occurs after 6 days of treatment, a platelet count should be performed 1 week after starting heparin treatment.

■ As experience with LMWHs in pregnancy has grown, the use of coagulation studies to monitor their use has fallen. Prophylactic doses of LMWH do not prolong the APTT, and no monitoring is required for these doses. Thrombocytopenia with LMWH is extremely rare.

■ Heparin levels, based on anti-Xa assays, can and should be monitored if LMWHs are being used to treat thrombosis in pregnancy. Peak anti-Xa levels

(3 hours postinjection) of 0.4–1.0 unit/ml are the aim. The assay must be calibrated for the particular heparin or LMWH in use.

■ Sadly, there is no way to predict which women will develop heparin-induced osteoporosis. Particular caution is needed in women taking concurrent corticosteroids or with known osteopenia/osteoporosis. The serum calcium level gives no indication of the bone stores of calcium.

■ Co-administration of calcium and vitamin D supplements (e.g. Calcichew D3 [12.5 mmol Ca + vit D 200 units] 2 tablets daily) may be considered for those whose dietary intake is low and who require long-term heparin in pregnancy.

Intrapartum management

■ Because of the high risk of thromboembolism immediately postpartum, heparin should not be discontinued during labour for longer than is necessary to allow safe regional anaesthesia or analgesia.

■ For those 'low-risk' women starting prophylaxis with heparin intrapartum, the first dose should ideally be administered prior to delivery.

■ Heparin in low/prophylactic doses does not interfere with the activation of normal haemostatic mechanisms at the site of injury, but only lowers the risk of spontaneous haemostatic activation. A coagulation screen and platelet count should be checked prior to siting of an epidural/spinal block. A normal screen indicates no extra risk of epidural haematoma.

■ In controlled studies, at least 10 000 patients have been given the combination of LMWH in prophylactic doses and epidural/spinal anaesthesia without complications. However, following the issue of an FDA warning regarding the risk of epidural haematoma with LMWH use (Clexane 30 mg b.d. in mostly elderly women undergoing orthopaedic surgery in the USA), most UK obstetric anaesthetists advise a 6–12-hour delay after the last LMWH injection before the siting of a regional block. LMWH can then be safely administered after about 2 hours.

■ The most vulnerable time for epidural haematomas seems to be after removal of the epidural catheter. Therefore this too should be in close collaboration with the obstetric anaesthetist and usually after a further 6–12-hour period after the last LMWH injection.

Postpartum management

■ Neither warfarin nor heparin is excreted in breast milk and breast-feeding is not contraindicated with use of these drugs.

■ The important principle is that for low- and high-risk women (Table 3.3), prophylaxis with either warfarin or s.c. heparin should be continued for 6 weeks after delivery.

- The advantages of changing to warfarin after the first week after delivery are that:
  - Exposure to heparin is minimised
  - There is no further need for self-administered s.c. injections.
- The disadvantages relate to the need for close monitoring, venepuncture, and attendance at an anticoagulation clinic.
- Women who have suffered a DVT or PE towards the end of their pregnancy, may require longer periods (e.g. 3 months) of warfarinisation postpartum.
- Women who have received more than 10–12 weeks' heparin therapy and who are deemed to be at high risk of osteoporosis may be offered postpartum bone densitometry. This is usually done by means of a dual X-ray absorptiometry (DEXA) scan, which compares the bone density of the spine and hip to the mean for age and sex-matched non-pregnant controls.

Thromboembolic disease in pregnancy – points to remember

- PE is the commonest cause of death in pregnancy and the puerperium in the UK.
- Pregnancy is associated with an increased risk of thrombosis.
- The risk of DVT and PE in pregnancy increases with increasing maternal age.
- Emergency caesarean section is associated with a greater than twenty-fold increase of dying from pulmonary embolism compared to spontaneous vaginal delivery.
- Objective diagnosis of DVT and PE is vital.
- Treatment is as for the non-pregnant patient, except that larger doses of i.v. heparin are often required and warfarin is avoided. There is less experience of treatment using LMWH.
- Some form of prophylaxis must be continued for the rest of the pregnancy and the puerperium.
- Long-term heparin use carries the risk of heparin-induced osteoporosis.
- Decisions regarding thromboprophylaxis in pregnancy relate to the past history and the presence of detectable thrombophilia.
- Women at high risk of recurrent thrombosis should receive antenatal, intrapartum and postnatal thromboprophylaxis.
- Heparin and warfarin are safe to use in lactating mothers.

Cerebral vein thrombosis

- Cerebral vein thrombosis (CVT) is uncommon (incidence approximately 1 in 10 000), but associated with a high mortality rate.
- The pregnant and puerperal state account for 5–20% (western Europe and USA) to 60% (India) of all cases of CVT.
- Most cases related to pregnancy occur in the puerperium. Six out of seven of the maternal deaths due to CVT in the UK during 1991–1996 occurred post-partum.

Clinical features

Patients usually present with the following symptoms:

- Headache
- Seizures
- Impaired consciousness
- Signs of raised intracranial pressure
- Vomiting
- Photophobia
- One-third to two-thirds of patients have focal signs such as hemiparesis. Focal signs depend on the territory of the thrombosis that may involve the cortical veins or the superior sagittal sinus
- CVT may cause fever and leukocytosis
- Venous infarction and intracerebral bleeding may result from obstruction of collateral circulation.

Pathogenesis

- This relates to the hypercoagulable postpartum state and possible trauma to the endothelial lining of cerebral sinuses and veins during labour.
- Puerperal infection and dehydration may explain the high incidence in developing countries.
- Many cases described are associated with thrombophilia.

Diagnosis

- Differential diagnosis includes eclampsia, subarachnoid haemorrhage, and herpes encephalitis.
- Diagnosis is made by computerised tomography (CT) scan to detect intracerebral bleeding, although magnetic resonance imaging (MRI), and especially venous angiography MRI, is best able to show venous clots.

Management

- This includes hydration, anticonvulsants, and anticoagulation.
- Treatment with heparin is controversial since the risk of intracerebral bleeding may be increased, but clot formation is prevented. Evidence mainly from non-pregnant patients suggests outcome is better with heparin therapy.
- A thrombophilia screen is mandatory. This is an unusual site for venous thrombosis and thrombophilia is found in a significant proportion of cases.

Further reading

Brill-Edwards, P., Ginsberg, J.S., Gent, M. et al. (2000) Safety of withholding heparin in pregnant women with a history of venous thromboembolism. *N. Engl. J. Med.*, **343,** 1439–1444.

Department of Health, Welsh Office, Scottish Home and Health Department and Department of Health and Social Services, Northern Ireland (1998) *Confidential Enquiries into Maternal Deaths in the United Kingdom 1994–96.* London: HMSO.

Ellison, J., Walker, I.D. and Greer, I.A. (2000) Antenatal use of enoxaparin for prevention and treatment of thromboembolism in pregnancy. *Br. J. Obstet. Gynaecol.*, **107,** 1116–1121.

Gerhardt, A., Scharf, R.E., Beckmann, M.W. et al. (2000) Prothrombin and factor V mutations in women with a history of thrombosis during pregnancy and the puerperium. *N. Engl. J. Med.*, **342,** 374–380.

Greer, I.A. (2000) The challenge of thrombophilia in maternal fetal medicine. *N. Engl. J. Med.*, **342,** 424–425.

Kupferminc, M.J., Eldor, A., Steinman, N. et al. (1999) Increased frequency of genetic thrombophilia in women with complications of pregnancy. *N. Engl. J. Med.*, **340,** 9–13.

McColl, M.D., Walker, I.D. and Greer, I.A. (1999) The role of inherited thrombophilia in venous thromboembolism associated with pregnancy. *Br. J. Obstet. Gynaecol.*, **106,** 756.

Nelson-Piercy, C. (1999) Thrombophilia and adverse pregnancy outcome: has the time come for routine testing? *Br. J. Obstet. Gynaecol.*, **106,** 513–515.

Nelson-Piercy, C., Letsky, E.A. and de Swiet, M. (1997) Low molecular weight heparin for obstetric thromboprophylaxis: experience of 69 pregnancies in 61 high risk women. *Am. J. Obstet. Gynecol.*, **176,** 1062–1068.

Powers, R.W., Minich, L.A., Lykins, D.L. et al. (1999) *J. Soc. Gynaecol. Investig.*, **6,** 74–79.

Royal College of Obstetricians and Gynaecologists (1995) *Thromboembolic Disease in Gynaecology and Pregnancy: Recommendations for Prophylaxis.* London: RCOG.

Sanson, B., Lensing, A.W.A., Prins, M.H. et al. (1999) Safety of low-molecular-weight heparin in pregnancy: A systematic review. *Thromb. Haemost.*, **81,** 668–672.

CHAPTER 4

Respiratory disease

Physiological changes	Tuberculosis
Asthma	Sarcoidosis
Hayfever	Cystic fibrosis
Pneumonia	Severe restrictive lung disease

Readers should also consult Section B for discussions on breathlessness (Table 1) and chest pain (Table 3).

Physiological changes

(Table 4.1)

■ There is a significant increase in oxygen demand in normal pregnancy. This is due to the increased metabolic rate and a 20% increased consumption of oxygen.

■ There is a 40–50% increase in minute ventilation, mostly due to an increase in tidal volume, rather than in respiratory rate.

■ This maternal hyperventilation causes arterial pO_2 to increase and arterial pCO_2 to fall, with a compensatory fall in serum bicarbonate to 18–22 mmol/l. A mild fully compensated respiratory alkalosis is therefore normal in pregnancy (arterial pH 7.44).

■ A potential source of diagnostic confusion is the increased awareness of the physiological hyperventilation of pregnancy leading to a subjective feeling of breathlessness in up to three-quarters of women at some time during pregnancy.

Asthma

Asthma is the commonest chronic medical illness to complicate pregnancy, affecting up to 7% of women of child-bearing age. It is often undiagnosed and when recognised, may be undertreated. Pregnancy provides an opportunity to diagnose asthma, and to optimise the treatment of women already known to have asthma.

Table 4.1 – Physiological changes in respiratory function during pregnancy

Physiological variable	Direction of change	Degree/timing of change
Oxygen consumption	↑	20%
Metabolic rate	↑	15%
Resting minute ventilation	↑	40–50%
Tidal volume	↑	
Respiratory rate	→	
Functional residual capacity	↓	Third trimester
Vital capacity	→	
FEV$_1$ and PEFR	→	
PaO$_2$	↑	
PaCO$_2$	↓	4.0 kPa/30 mmHg
Arterial pH	↑	7.44

FEV$_1$: forced expiratory volume in 1 second; PEFR: peak expiratory flow rate; ↑: increased; ↓: decreased; →: unchanged.

Clinical features

Symptoms

- Cough
- Breathlessness
- Wheezy breathing
- Chest tightness.

Symptoms are commonly worse at night and in the early morning. There may be clear provoking trigger factors, such as:

- Pollen
- Animal dander
- Exercise
- Emotion
- Upper respiratory tract infections.

Signs

Signs are often absent unless seen during an acute attack.

- Increased respiratory rate
- Inability to complete sentences
- Wheeze
- Use of accessory muscles
- Tachycardia.

Pathogenesis

Reversible bronchoconstriction is caused by the following:

- Smooth-muscle spasm in the airway walls
- Inflammation with swelling and excessive production of mucus.

Diagnosis

- This is made by eliciting a history of typical symptoms.
- It is the variability and reversibility of the obstruction rather than the absolute level that is important when considering a diagnosis of asthma.
- A typical sign is morning 'dipping' in the peak flow.
- The degree of bronchoconstriction is measured with a peak expiratory flow rate (PEFR) or forced expiratory volume in 1 second (FEV_1). Greater than 15% improvement in these parameters following inhalation of a β-sympathomimetic bronchodilator is diagnostic.

Pregnancy

Effect of pregnancy on asthma

- Asthma may improve, deteriorate or remain unchanged during pregnancy.
- Women with only mild disease are unlikely to experience problems, whereas severe asthmatics are at greater risk of deterioration, particularly late in pregnancy.
- Those women whose symptoms improve during the last trimester of pregnancy may experience postnatal deterioration.
- Deterioration in disease control is commonly caused by reduction or even complete cessation of medication due to fears about its safety.

Effect of asthma on pregnancy

- In most women there are no adverse effects of asthma on pregnancy outcome.
- Severe, poorly controlled asthma, associated with chronic or intermittent

maternal hypoxaemia, may adversely affect the fetus.

- Some association (mostly from retrospective, uncontrolled or small studies) between maternal asthma and the following:
  - Pregnancy-induced hypertension/pre-eclampsia
  - Preterm births and premature labour
  - Low-birthweight infants
  - Intrauterine growth restriction (IUGR)
  - Neonatal morbidity, for example:
    - Transient tachypnoea of the newborn
    - Neonatal hypoglycaemia
    - Neonatal seizures
    - Admission to the neonatal intensive care unit.
- In general, adverse effects on pregnancy outcome are small and related to the severity and control of the asthma.
- None of the above associations are common in clinical practice.
- Women should be advised that their asthma is unlikely to adversely affect their pregnancy and maintaining good control of asthma throughout pregnancy may minimise any small risks.

Management

- Current emphasis in the management of asthma is on the prevention, rather than the treatment, of acute attacks.
- It is important to check the inhaler technique of the patient, since failure to do this may result in unnecessary escalation of therapy. Some women require a breath-actuated inhaler.
- Regular inhaled anti-inflammatory medication is considered first-line maintenance treatment for all but those with infrequent symptoms.
- If usage of a 'reliever' (β_2-agonist) inhaler exceeds >once/day, a 'preventer' (beclomethasone) inhaler should be commenced.
- The aim of treatment is to achieve virtual total freedom from symptoms, such that the lifestyle of the individual is not affected. Regrettably, many people with asthma accept chronic symptoms such as wheezing or 'chest tightness' on waking as an inevitable consequence of their disease. This is inappropriate and pregnancy provides an ideal opportunity to educate women with asthma, taking into account the following guidelines:
  - Asthmatics should be encouraged to avoid known trigger factors.
  - Home peak-flow monitoring and personalised self-management plans should be encouraged.
  - An increase in the dose or frequency of an inhaled steroid should be the first step if symptoms are not optimally controlled on the current dose. This should be administered via a large volume spacer.

– Women should be counselled about indications for an increase in inhaled steroid dosage and if appropriate given an 'emergency' supply of oral steroids.

The treatment of asthma in pregnancy is essentially no different from the treatment of asthma in non-pregnant women. All the drugs in widespread use to treat asthma, including systemic steroids, appear to be safe in pregnancy and during lactation. The challenge in the management of pregnant asthmatics is to ensure adequate preconceptual or early pregnancy counselling so that women do not stop important anti-inflammatory inhaled therapy. Strong and repeated reassurance regarding the importance and safety of regular medication is needed to ensure compliance.

Medication

Corticosteroids

Use of both inhaled and oral steroids is safe in pregnancy. Only minimal amounts of inhaled corticosteroid preparations are systemically absorbed. There is no evidence for an increased incidence of congenital malformations or adverse fetal effects attributable to the use of inhaled beclomethasone (Becotide®) or budesonide (Pulmicort®). Fluticasone propionate (Flixotide®) is a newer inhaled corticosteroid that may be used for those requiring high doses of inhaled steroids.

The addition of systemic corticosteroids to control exacerbations of asthma is safe, and these must not be withheld if current medications are inadequate.

Prednisolone is metabolised by the placenta, and very little (10%) active drug reaches the fetus. Findings of an increased incidence of cleft palate in the offspring of rabbits treated with massive doses of cortisone early in gestation have been wrongly extrapolated to human pregnancy. There is no evidence of an increased risk of abortion, stillbirth, congenital malformations, or neonatal death attributable to maternal steroid therapy.

Although suppression of the fetal hypothalamic–pituitary–adrenal axis is a theoretical possibility with maternal systemic steroid therapy, there is little evidence from clinical practice to support this.

Long-term, high-dose steroids may increase the risk of premature rupture of the membranes.

There have been more recent concerns regarding the potential adverse effects of steroid exposure *in utero* (such as from repeated high-dose i.m. steroids to induce fetal lung maturation) and neurodevelopmental problems in the child. More work is needed before such concerns can be extrapolated to the use of oral steroids for medical disorders in the mother.

Oral steroids will increase the risk of gestational diabetes, and cause deterioration in blood–glucose control in women with established impairment of glucose tolerance in pregnancy. Blood glucose should be checked regularly; the hyperglycaemia is amenable to treatment with diet and, if required, insulin, and is reversible on cessation or reduction of steroid dose. The development of hyper-glycaemia is not an indication to discontinue or decrease the dose of oral steroids, the requirement for which must be determined by the asthma.

β_2-agonists

β_2-agonists from the systemic circulation cross the placenta rapidly, but very little of a given inhaled dose reaches the lungs, and only a minute fraction of this reaches the systemic circulation. Studies show no difference in perinatal mortality, congenital malformations, birthweight, Apgar scores or delivery complications when pregnant asthmatics treated with inhaled β_2-agonists are compared with asthmatics not using β_2-agonists and non-asthmatic controls. Experience with the use of the inhaled long-acting β_2-agonist, salmeterol (Serevent®) in pregnancy is growing and it too appears to be safe. It should not be discontinued in pregnant asthmatics who require it for good asthma control.

No adverse fetal effects have been reported with the use of the following drugs:

- Inhaled disodium cromoglycate (Intal®)
- Inhaled nedocromil (Tilade®)
- Inhaled anticholinergic drugs (e.g. Atrovent®).

Methylxanthines

These are no longer recommended as first-line treatment of asthma, but have been used extensively in the past. In those few women who are dependent on therapeutic levels of theophylline, the dose may need to be increased in pregnancy. Such increases should be guided by drug levels. Both theophylline and aminophylline readily cross the placenta and fetal theophylline levels are similar to those of the mother. In large studies, the incidence of congenital malformations in women receiving theophylline during the first trimester is not significantly higher than that in asthmatic or non-asthmatic controls. Theophylline has been shown to be a cardiovascular teratogen in animals, and one report has suggested a possible link between theophylline and three cases of congenital cardiac anomalies in the human. There is no conclusive evidence of ill effect or malformation in the human fetus. Some studies have noted transient tachycardia, jaundice or irritability in neonates of mothers receiving xanthines, but this may relate to disease severity rather than the drug itself.

Low-dose aspirin

It is important to consider the possibility of 'aspirin sensitivity' and severe bronchospasm in a minority of women with asthma. Low-dose aspirin may be indicated in pregnancy as prophylaxis for certain women at high risk of early-onset pre-eclampsia (see chapter 1), antiphospholipid syndrome (see chapter 8), migraine prophylaxis (chapter 9) or thromboprophylaxis (see chapter 3). Pregnant asthmatic women should be asked about a history of aspirin sensitivity before being advised to take low-dose aspirin.

Acute severe asthma

- Acute severe attacks of asthma are dangerous and should be vigorously managed in hospital. The treatment is no different from the emergency management of acute severe asthma in the non-pregnant woman.
- These patients require i.v. rehydration, oxygen, and β_2-agonists that should be administered via a nebuliser using oxygen and not air, and in repeated doses if necessary. A chest X-ray should be performed if there is any clinical suspicion of pneumonia or pneumothorax, or if the woman fails to improve.
- If the PEFR does not improve to >70% predicted, the woman should be admitted to hospital. If she is discharged, this must be with a tapering course of oral steroids and arrangements for review.
- Steroids are more likely to be withheld from pregnant than non-pregnant asthmatics presenting via Accident and Emergency departments. This is inappropriate and leads to an increase in ongoing exacerbation of asthma.
- Those admitted to hospital also require oral or i.v. steroids; in severe cases i.v. aminophylline or i.v. β_2-agonists should be used as indicated. Sudden severe deterioration or failure to respond to treatment should raise the possibility of a pneumothorax or pulmonary embolus.

Intrapartum management

- Asthmatic attacks in labour are exceedingly rare. Women should not discontinue their prophylactic inhalers during labour, and there is no evidence to suggest that β_2-agonists given via the inhaled route impair uterine contraction or delay the onset of labour.
- Women receiving oral steroids (prednisolone >7.5 mg/day for >2 weeks prior to delivery), should receive parenteral hydrocortisone (100 mg three or four times/day) to cover the stress of labour, and until oral medication is restarted.
- Prostaglandin E2, used to induce labour, to ripen the cervix, or for early termination of pregnancy, is a bronchodilator and is safe to use.
- The use of prostaglandin F2α to treat life-threatening postpartum haemorrhage may be unavoidable, but it can cause bronchospasm and should be used with caution in asthmatics.
- All forms of pain relief in labour, including epidural analgesia and Entonox can be used safely by asthmatic women, although in the unlikely event of an acute severe asthmatic attack, opiates for pain relief should be avoided.

Epidural, rather than general anaesthesia, is preferable because of the decreased risk of chest infection and atelectasis.

■ Ergometrine has been reported to cause bronchospasm, in particular in association with general anaesthesia, but this does not seem to be a practical problem when Syntometrine (oxytocin and ergometrine) is used for the prophylaxis of postpartum haemorrhage.

Asthma – points to remember

■ Pregnancy itself does not usually influence the severity of asthma.

■ For the majority of women, asthma has no adverse effect on pregnancy outcome, and women should be reassured accordingly.

■ Poorly controlled severe asthma presents more of a risk to the pregnancy than the medication used to prevent or treat it. This small risk is minimised with good control.

■ Education and reassurance, ideally prior to conception, concerning the safety of asthma medications during pregnancy are integral parts of management.

■ Decreasing or stopping inhaled anti-inflammatory therapy during pregnancy is a frequent cause of potentially dangerous deterioration in disease control.

■ Inhaled, oral and i.v. steroids and inhaled, nebulised and i.v. β_2-agonists are safe to use in pregnancy and while breast-feeding.

■ Treatment of asthma in pregnancy differs little from the management in the non-pregnant patient. Effective control of the disease process and its accompanying symptoms is a priority.

■ An increase in the dose or frequency of inhaled steroids should be the first step if symptoms are not optimally controlled on the current dose of inhaled steroids and the inhaler technique is good.

Breast-feeding

■ The risk of atopic disease developing in the child of an asthmatic woman is about 1 in 10, or 1 in 3 if both parents are atopic. There is some evidence that breast-feeding may reduce this risk. This may be a result of the delay in the introduction of cows' milk protein.

■ All the drugs discussed above, including oral steroids, are safe to use in breast-feeding mothers.

■ Prednisolone is secreted in breast milk, but there have been no reported adverse clinical effects in infants breast-fed by mothers receiving prednisolone. Concerns regarding neonatal adrenal function are unwarranted with doses below 30 mg/day.

Hayfever

Pregnant women should be reassured that there is no evidence to suggest that the drugs used to treat hayfever and allergic rhinitis, such as intranasal beclomethasone (Beconase®), and non-sedating antihistamines (terfenadine, Triludan®; astemizole, Hismanal®) are harmful to the fetus, and that these drugs may be used during pregnancy if required for control of symptoms.

Pneumonia

- Bacterial pneumonia is no more common in pregnant than in non-pregnant women of the same age, matched for smoking status.
- Viral pneumonia, for example influenza pneumonia, is more severe in pregnancy.
- Pregnant women are particularly susceptible to varicella-zoster (chickenpox) pneumonia.

Clinical features

Symptoms

- Cough (often dry at first)
- Fever
- Rigors
- Breathlessness
- Pleuritic pain.

Signs

- Fever
- Purulent sputum
- Coarse crackles on auscultation
- Signs of consolidation.

Pathogenesis

Bacterial

- *Streptococcus pneumoniae* (causative organism in >50% cases)

- *Haemophilus influenzae* (more common in chronic bronchitis)
- *Staphylococcus* (associated with influenza, i.v. drug abuse)
- *Legionella* (institutional outbreaks).

Viral

- Influenza A virus
- Varicella-zoster.

Atypical

- *Mycoplasma pneumoniae* (community acquired)
- *Pneumocystis carinii* (in association with HIV).

Diagnosis

- Diagnosis may be delayed if there is reluctance to perform a chest X-ray.
- The ionising radiation from a chest X-ray is approximately 0.2 rad (less than 1/20th of the maximum recommended exposure in pregnancy, i.e. 5 rad) and abdominal shielding will minimise the exposure to the fetus.
- If a chest X-ray is clinically indicated, this investigation must not be withheld.
- A sputum culture should be taken.
- Bacterial pneumonia is associated with a raised white blood cell (WBC) count.
- Mycoplasma pneumonia does not usually cause a raised WBC count, but is associated with cold agglutinins in 50% of cases and may be diagnosed by a rising antibody titre.
- If the patient is breathless, an analysis of arterial blood gases should be performed. Profound hypoxia out of proportion to the chest X-ray findings should alert the clinician to the possibility of *Pneumocystis* infection.
- If the woman fails to respond to conventional antibiotics, a search for non-bacterial causes of pneumonia should be made with serology for *Mycoplasma*, and possibly bronchoscopy if a diagnosis of *Pneumocystis* infection is suspected.

Management

The principles are as follows:

- Maintain adequate oxygenation. Monitor with oximetry and administer oxygen if hypoxic.
- Maintain adequate hydration. The woman is likely to be dehydrated, especially if there is fever.

- Administer physiotherapy to help clear secretions.
- Direct chemotherapy at the causative organism:
- Management of bacterial pneumonia in pregnancy should follow the guidelines for treatment in the non-pregnant woman:
  - For most cases of community-acquired pneumonia, amoxycillin and erythromycin are the appropriate antibiotics.
  - Cephalosporins should be used for hospital-acquired infection.
  - Tetracyclines should be avoided after about 20 weeks' gestation since they can cause discolouration of the teeth in the fetus.
  - Clearance of renally excreted drugs increases in pregnancy and therefore higher doses (e.g. amoxycillin 500 mg t.d.s.) are required.

Varicella

- Chickenpox is highly infectious and most children become infected.
- The incubation period is 14–21 days and the period of infectivity is from 1 day prior to eruption of the rash to 6 days after the rash disappears.
- Chickenpox is more severe in adults, and pregnant women are particularly susceptible to varicella pneumonia, for which the maternal and fetal mortality rates are high.
- Infection occurs in 0.05–0.07% of pregnancies and about 10–20% of infected women develop varicella pneumonia.
- A history of previous infection and therefore likely immunity is usually reliable in the case of chickenpox since the clinical features are so unique. Serology can be checked.
- A live attenuated vaccine has recently become available in the USA and should be offered to non-immune women preconception.
- Because of the substantial risk accompanying chickenpox infection in pregnancy, non-immune pregnant women exposed to varicella should be given zoster immunoglobulin (ZIG).
- Women should be asked about previous chickenpox infection before they are prescribed steroids in pregnancy, and those found not to be immune given ZIG.
- Those women who do develop clinical varicella should be treated with acyclovir. The oral formulation is safe in pregnancy, but caution is needed when using i.v. acyclovir in pregnancy.
- Anyone with varicella should be examined at a distance from the antenatal clinic to minimise exposure to other pregnant women.
- Maternal and neonatal morbidity and mortality in cases of maternal varicella pneumonia justifies the use of i.v. acyclovir.
- A study has suggested that later gestational age (perhaps because of increased immunosuppression) at the onset of varicella pneumonia is a significant risk factor for maternal mortality.

■ The fetus is at risk of congenital varicella with maternal infection in the first 12–16 weeks of pregnancy. The risk of teratogenicity is about 2%.

■ Detailed ultrasound scanning should be offered at 16–20 weeks' gestation or 5 weeks after infection, whichever is sooner. The most common abnormalities are dermatomal skin scarring, eye defects, limb hypoplasia and neurological abnormalities.

■ There is a risk of neonatal varicella if infection occurs within 10 days of delivery. If practical, delivery should be delayed until 5–7 days after the onset of maternal illness to allow passive transfer of antibodies. If delivery occurs within 5 days of maternal infection or if the mother develops chickenpox within 2 days of giving birth, the neonate should receive ZIG. This does not prevent all cases of neonatal infection, which may be fatal (30% mortality rate).

Pneumonia – points to remember

■ Chest X-rays are safe to use in pregnancy.

■ Most antibiotics are safe to use in pregnancy and during lactation; caution is required with aminoglycosides and tetracycline.

■ A higher dose (500 mg t.d.s.) of amoxycillin is required in pregnancy.

■ Varicella pneumonia may be fatal in pregnancy and active steps must be taken to prevent chickenpox infection in pregnancy.

■ Non-immune pregnant women exposed to varicella or prescribed steroids in pregnancy should be given ZIG.

■ If a pregnant woman does contract chickenpox, she should be treated with acyclovir as soon as possible.

Pneumocystis carinii pneumonia (PCP)

■ The increasing number of women of child-bearing age who are seropositive for human immunodeficiency virus (HIV) has contributed to the increased incidence of pneumonia in pregnancy.

■ The most common opportunistic infection in patients progressing to acquired immune deficiency syndrome (AIDS) is PCP.

■ PCP is associated with adverse obstetric outcome, particularly if the diagnosis is not suspected.

■ PCP should be treated with high-dose trimethoprim-sulphamethoxazole (co-trimoxazole [Septrin]) with or without pentamidine.

■ Despite the theoretical risks of neonatal kernicterus or haemolysis from sulphonamides given at term, there is increasing evidence that Septrin use is safe in pregnancy. Indeed, PCP is one of the remaining indications for the use of Septrin. In practice it is only long-acting sulphonamides such as sulphadimidine that have ever been shown to affect the binding of bilirubin in the fetus or neonate.

■ Because PCP is an important cause of AIDS-related maternal mortality, HIV-infected pregnant women with a history of this opportunistic infection or with a CD4+ cell count of <200 cells/μl should receive prophylaxis with either Septrin or nebulised pentamidine.

(See also HIV infection in pregnancy, chapter 15).

Tuberculosis (TB)

■ Rates of TB are increasing in the UK, Europe, the USA and developing countries.

■ This recent resurgence is partly due to the susceptibility of HIV-infected patients to tuberculosis infection.

■ In the UK and the USA there are reports of increasing rates among the homeless and in inner-city populations. In New York, USA, rates of pulmonary TB in pregnant women increased almost eight-fold between 1985 and 1992.

■ In the UK it is more common in Asian and West Indian immigrants.

Clinical features

Symptoms

The onset is usually insidious and symptoms include:

■ Cough
■ Haemoptysis
■ Weight loss (or failure to gain weight)
■ Night sweats.

Signs

■ TB can cause almost any chest signs.
■ It most typically affects the upper lobes, with coarse crackles, dullness on percussion over the clavicle, or in advanced or old cases, signs of fibrosis with deviation of the trachea towards the side of the infection.
■ Signs of associated lymphadenopathy, and erythema nodosum (see also p. 243).

Pathogenesis

- Causative organism is *Mycobacterium tuberculosis* (MBTB).
- *Mycobacterium avium-intracellulare* is an important cause of pulmonary infection in AIDS patients.

Diagnosis

- This is suggested by the typical appearances on a chest X-ray.
- Diagnosis is confirmed by sputum examination for acid-fast bacilli (Ziehl–Neelsen stain).
- Culture of the organism takes about 6 weeks.
- If there is no sputum, washings from bronchoscopy must be obtained.
- The Mantoux test (0.1 ml of 10 tuberculin units of purified protein derivative of MBTB) is not affected by pregnancy but is rarely used since it cannot differentiate between a past infection and active disease.

Pregnancy

Effect of pregnancy on tuberculosis

- There is little evidence to suggest that TB has a detrimental effect on pregnancy or that pregnancy adversely affects disease progression in patients receiving, or who have received, effective antituberculous therapy.
- Congenital TB with infection via the umbilical vein or amniotic fluid is rare. Neonatal TB via airborne inoculation from the infected mother with active but undiagnosed or untreated TB is important in developing countries.

Management

- The principles of management are similar in pregnant and non-pregnant patients.
- Untreated TB represents a greater hazard to pregnant women and their fetuses than the treatment itself.
- The advice of a respiratory physician must be sought and pregnant mothers with TB should be treated without delay.
- Active disease should be treated with a prolonged supervised course of more than one drug to which the organism is sensitive. Before sensitivities are available, most patients are given triple/quadruple therapy with:
  - Rifampicin (liver function tests should be monitored regularly)
  - Isoniazid
  - Pyrazinamide and/or ethambutol.

Potential risk to the fetus of antituberculous chemotherapy

- Ethambutol and isoniazid are safe to use in pregnancy, but all patients taking isoniazid should also be prescribed pyridoxine 50 mg/day to reduce the risk of peripheral neuritis. Liver function should be monitored monthly because of the risk of isoniazid-related hepatotoxicity.
- Although there have been concerns regarding a teratogenic risk with rifampicin, no adverse fetal effects have yet been proven.
- Streptomycin has been associated with a high (>10%) incidence of eighth nerve damage and should therefore be avoided throughout pregnancy.
- There are limited data concerning the safety of pyrazinamide in pregnancy, and therefore it is best avoided until the completion of organogenesis.

Postnatal care

- The mother usually becomes non-infectious within 2 weeks of beginning treatment.
- If the mother is sputum positive, the risk of the neonate developing active TB is high unless prophylactic treatment with isoniazid (assuming the mother's organism is isoniazid sensitive) is given.
- The baby should also be given bacille Calmette–Guérin (BCG). As isoniazid does not impair the immunogenicity of the BCG vaccine, there is no benefit in using isoniazid-resistant strains of BCG for combined prophylaxis.
- The amounts of antituberculous drugs excreted in breast milk are only a fraction of the usual therapeutic dose and are not sufficient to dissuade women from breast-feeding.

Tuberculosis – points to remember

- TB is particularly common in Asian immigrants.
- Perform a chest X-ray if TB is suspected.
- Seek the advice of a respiratory physician.
- Diagnosis must be confirmed bacteriologically, which may necessitate bronchoscopy.
- Give BCG to the neonate and isoniazid in high-risk cases.

Sarcoidosis

Sarcoidosis is uncommon in pregnancy, perhaps affecting 0.05% of all pregnancies in the UK.

Clinical features

- There may be chest symptoms, but the patient is often asymptomatic.
- Extrapulmonary manifestations include:
  - Erythema nodosum (may also occur as an isolated finding in pregnancy without evidence of an underlying associated cause) (see also chapter 13, p. 243)
  - Anterior uveitis
  - Hypercalcaemia
  - Arthropathy
  - Fever
  - Central nervous system (CNS) involvement.

Pathogenesis

- Sarcoidosis is a multi-system granulomatous disorder of unknown aetiology.
- Unlike tuberculosis, the granulomata are non-caseating.

Diagnosis

- Chest X-ray. The commonest feature is bilateral hilar lymphadenopathy. There may be extensive pulmonary infiltration progressing to fibrosis.
- Although there may be no obvious infiltration in the lung fields, the lung parenchyma is usually involved and diagnosis is made by bronchoalveolar lavage and transbronchial biopsy.
- Serum levels of angiotensin-converting enzyme (ACE) may be altered in normal pregnancy and cannot therefore be used to help diagnosis or monitor disease activity as in the non-pregnant patient.

Effect of pregnancy on sarcoidosis

- The course of the disease may be unaffected or improved by pregnancy.
- Those with active disease may have resolution of their X-ray changes during pregnancy and there is a tendency for sarcoidosis to relapse in the puerperium.
- Any improvement that is seen antenatally may be due to the increased levels of endogenous cortisol present in pregnancy.

Management

- Sarcoidosis often resolves spontaneously, but indications for steroid treatment include the following:

- Extrapulmonary, especially CNS, disease
- Functional respiratory impairment.

■ The safety of steroids in pregnancy has been discussed earlier (see under 'Asthma', p. 63), and they should be continued or started in pregnancy if clinically indicated.

■ As with asthmatics on maintenance steroids, labour and delivery should be covered with parenteral hydrocortisone if women are taking >7.5 mg daily of prednisolone (see p. 65).

■ Women should be advised not to take supplemental vitamin D, which may precipitate hypercalcaemia in patients with sarcoidosis.

Sarcoidosis – points to remember

■ Erythema nodosum may occur in a normal pregnancy.
■ The course of sarcoidosis is unaltered or improved by pregnancy.
■ Use systemic steroids if indicated.
■ Consider a prophylactic increase in steroid dose postpartum.
■ Serum ACE is not useful in pregnancy.
■ Avoid vitamin D.

Cystic fibrosis

Increasing numbers of children with cystic fibrosis (CF) are surviving into adulthood. Males are usually sterile, but female fertility, especially in the well nourished, is normal.

Clinical features

■ Chronic lung infection, bronchiectasis, respiratory failure
■ Pancreatic insufficiency leading to malnutrition and diabetes
■ The median age at death for CF patients is now about 30 years.

Pathogenesis

■ CF is due to a dysfunction of all exocrine glands with abnormal mucus production and high sweat sodium.
■ It is the commonest autosomal recessive disorder in the UK, with a carrier rate of 1 in 25.

- Although a specific mutation on chromosome 7 has been identified, not all patients with CF have the deletion and patients with CF are heterogeneous and include different genetic errors or altered penetration.

- CF is caused by abnormalities in the CF transmembrane conductance regulator protein, a transmembranous chloride channel, causing impaired hydration of secretions in glandular organs.

- Gene therapy offers the potential of a more effective approach to the treatment of CF, but although clinical trials are in progress, this has yet to become a routine option in CF patients.

Pregnancy

Effect of pregnancy on CF

- Most patients with CF die in early adult life, but with few exceptions (see later) pregnancy does not increase this risk.

- Maternal mortality is significantly increased compared with normal pregnant women.

- Maternal mortality is not significantly greater than non-pregnant age-matched women with cystic fibrosis.

- Pregnancy is well tolerated by most mothers with CF (perhaps because those who survive and become pregnant have a less severe form of the disease).

- Mortality is increased in women with moderate to severe lung disease (FEV_1 <60% predicted) at the onset of pregnancy and maternal survival is positively correlated with pre-pregnancy % FEV_1.

- Other adverse factors on maternal disease are similar to those that adversely affect fetal morbidity and mortality (see later), namely maternal pulmonary hypertension, cyanosis and hypoxaemia.

- Women may deteriorate and die while the child is still young and it is important that such issues are discussed with the women and their partners prior to pregnancy.

The main maternal morbidity in CF pregnancies is as follows:

- Poor maternal weight gain. Even those without pancreatic insufficiency are often underweight at the onset of pregnancy and have difficulty gaining weight during pregnancy.

- Deterioration in lung function with worsening dyspnoea, exercise tolerance and oxygen saturation. Although there is usually loss of lung function during pregnancy, this is regained following delivery.

- Pulmonary infective exacerbations.

- Congestive cardiac failure.

Effect of CF on pregnancy

- The rate of spontaneous abortion is not increased in CF pregnancies.
- Despite the frequent use of high doses of antibiotics in these women, the rate of congenital abnormalities is not increased.
- Factors predicting a poor obstetric outcome include:
  - Pulmonary hypertension
  - Cyanosis
  - Arterial hypoxaemia (oxygen saturation <90%)
  - Moderate-to-severe lung disease (FEV_1 <60% predicted)
  - Poor maternal nutrition.

The commonest complications during pregnancy are:

- Prematurity (the preterm (<37 weeks) delivery rate is 30–50%).
- Intrauterine growth restriction. Chronic hypoxia (oxygen saturation <90%) and/or cyanosis increase the risk of small-for-gestational-age infants. Birth-weight is positively correlated with pre-pregnancy lung function (probably related to longer gestations).

Women with preserved pancreatic function have improved pregnancy outcome. Poor maternal weight gain is predictive of both prematurity and stillbirth.

Pre-pregnancy counselling

- This is essential. Pregnancy is safe in mild disease with FEV_1 >70–80% predicted but the following are contraindications to pregnancy:
  - Pulmonary hypertension
  - Cor pulmonale
  - FEV_1 <50% predicted
- Since *Burkholderia* cepacia may be associated with rapid deterioration in lung function, recent acquisition or declining lung function in the presence of this organism may also be a contraindication to pregnancy.
- Screening for diabetes should be undertaken.
- Since all women with CF are homozygous, all offspring will be carriers of the CF gene.
- Determination of the carrier status of the partner. The risk of a child being born with CF is 2–2.5% if the carrier status of the father is unknown (based on a carrier rate in the general UK population of about 1 in 25), and 50% if the father is heterozygous for the gene.

Management

During pregnancy women with CF should be jointly managed in a CF centre and a specialist obstetric unit with experience in the management of such women.

Medical management during pregnancy should include attention to the following:

- Adequate maternal nutrition
- Control of pulmonary infection
- Avoidance of prolonged hypoxia
- Regular assessment of fetal growth.

Nutrition

- Of adult CF patients, over 90% have pancreatic insufficiency and require enzyme supplements. High-calorie dietary supplements may be required in order to maintain maternal weight, since patients with CF (even without malabsorption) have high energy requirements that will be further increased by pregnancy.
- Of adult CF patients, 20% have diabetes and a further 15% have impaired glucose tolerance (IGT). Insulin requirements increase in pregnancy and those with IGT will be at risk of gestational diabetes (see p. 92).

Control of pulmonary infection

- Obsessional adherence to chest physiotherapy regimes must be encouraged. Some women decrease their physiotherapy due to fears concerning the fetus. These fears should be allayed.
- Most of the older, more established antibiotics used to treat pulmonary infective exacerbations in CF have a good safety record in pregnancy. Appropriate caution is needed when considering the use of new drugs for which there is little information in pregnancy. The risks to the fetus from poor maternal health probably outweigh the risks to the fetus from transplacental passage of drugs.
- Some patients may be taking prophylactic antibiotics either orally or via a nebuliser. Except in the case of tetracycline, which is contraindicated in pregnancy because of effects on fetal teeth and skeleton, these should usually be continued throughout pregnancy.
- Infective exacerbations should be treated aggressively and this is likely to require admission and i.v. penicillins and aminoglycosides, or cephalosporins in cases of resistant *Pseudomonas*.
- Antibiotic therapy must be dictated by the results of sputum cultures.
- Caution is needed when using i.v. aminoglycosides in pregnancy and regular monitoring of drug levels is required.

Some patients with CF exhibit reversibility in response to bronchodilators, and women should be reassured that inhaled and nebulised corticosteroids are safe for use in pregnancy (see p. 63).

Avoidance of prolonged hypoxia and timing of delivery

- Towards the middle and end of the third trimester, women with CF often become increasingly breathless, often without any obvious infective exacerbation.
- If there is resting hypoxia, and especially if oxygen saturation (%) is in the 80s or low 90s, admission for bed rest and oxygen therapy is advised.
- In some women, symptom deterioration warrants early delivery.
- The fetus is at risk of growth restriction and therefore the mother should be offered growth scans throughout pregnancy.
- If the growth rate slows, it may sometimes be improved by admission of the mother for bed rest, nutritional supplements and oxygen.
- In most cases, CF women deliver vaginally at term.
- Caesarean section is only necessary for obstetric indications and general anaesthesia should be avoided if possible.
- Instrumental delivery may be indicated to avoid a prolonged second stage.
- Patients with CF are particularly prone to pneumothoraces, which may be precipitated by prolonged attempts at pushing and repeated Valsalva manoeuvres in the second stage of labour.
- Breast-feeding should usually be encouraged, although the mother may continue to require nutritional supplements in the puerperium, especially if she is breast-feeding. Most of the drugs used will be secreted into the breast milk, but this is rarely a contraindication to breast-feeding.

Cystic fibrosis – points to remember

- Joint care should be maintained with a CF centre.
- Outcome is related to pre-pregnancy lung function.
- Perinatal outcome is usually good.
- Prematurity rates are high.
- Maternal outcome is variable.
- Specialist dietary advice with additional energy supplements should be given.
- Infective exacerbations should be treated aggressively.
- There is a risk of gestational diabetes.
- Induction of labour/early delivery may be necessary for relief of maternal symptoms.

Severe restrictive lung disease

■ Patients with severe lung disease are less likely to deteriorate in pregnancy than those with severe cardiac disease; this is because there is greater reserve in respiratory function than in cardiac function. Thus, although there is a comparative (about 40%) increase in both cardiac output and minute ventilation in pregnancy, for minute ventilation this represents a smaller fraction of the maximum increase achievable by the body.

■ It is difficult to predict with any accuracy the minimal forced vital capacity (FVC) compatible with successful pregnancy outcome in patients with kyphoscoliosis, scleroderma (see p. 151) and other causes of severe restrictive lung disease. Although figures such as 1 l or 50% of predicted FVC have been suggested, women with more severe impairment have had successful pregnancies.

■ Polycythaemia gives an indirect assessment of the degree of hypoxia and in itself is associated with an increased risk of thrombosis due to hyperviscosity.

■ Women with kyphoscoliosis are often delivered prematurely due to deterioration in respiratory function in the third trimester, and by caesarean section because of associated abnormalities of the bony pelvis and of abnormal presentations of the fetus.

■ Each case must be assessed individually. Whatever the underlying cause of respiratory insufficiency, significant hypercapnia or hypoxia, and pulmonary hypertension and cor pulmonale are associated with less favourable pregnancy outcomes.

Severe restrictive lung disease – points to remember

■ Women with severe lung disease are better able to tolerate pregnancy than women with severe cardiac insufficiency.

■ If the FVC is >1 l, a successful pregnancy is usually possible.

■ Respiratory diseases complicated by pulmonary hypertension and cor pulmonale have a poor prognosis in pregnancy.

Further reading

British Thoracic Society. The British Guidelines on Asthma Management (1997) 1995 review and position statement. *Thorax*, **52** (Suppl.) S1–S21.

Brown, Z.A. and Baker, D.A. (1989) Acyclovir therapy during pregnancy. *Obstet. Gynecol.*, **73** (3, part 2), 526–531.

Czeizel, A.E. and Rockenbauer, M. (1997) Population-based case-control study of teratogenic potential of corticosteroids. *Teratology*, **56,** 335–340.

Edenborough, F.P., Mackenzie, W.E. and Stableforth, D.E. (2000) The outcome of 72 pregnancies in 55 women with cystic fibrosis in the United Kingdom 1977–1996. *Br. J. Obstet. Gynaecol.*, **107**, 254–261.

Geddes, D.M. (1992) Cystic fibrosis and pregnancy. *J. Roy. Soc. Med.*, **85** (Suppl. 19), 36–37.

Jana, N., Ghosh, K., Sinha, S., Gopalan, S. and Vasishta, K. (1996) The perinatal aspects of pulmonary tuberculosis. *Fetal Maternal Med. Rev.*, **8**, 229–238.

Nelson-Piercy, C. (2001) Asthma during pregnancy. *Thorax*, 2001; **56**, 325–328.

Royal College of Obstetricians and Gynaecologists, UK (1997) Chicken pox in pregnancy. Notes:http//www.rcog.org.uk/guidelines/chicken_pox.html.

Schatz, M. (1999) Asthma and pregnancy. *Lancet*, **353**, 1202–1204.

Snider, D.E. (1984) Pregnancy and tuberculosis. *Chest*, **86** (Suppl.): 10S–13S.

CHAPTER 5
Diabetes

Physiological changes   Pre-existing diabetes

Gestational diabetes

Physiological changes

- Pregnancy, especially the last trimester, is a state of physiological insulin resistance and relative glucose intolerance.

- Glucose handling is significantly altered in pregnancy; fasting levels of glucose are decreased and serum levels following a meal or glucose load are increased compared to the non-pregnant state.

- Glucose tolerance decreases progressively with increasing gestation; this is largely due to the anti-insulin hormones secreted by the placenta in normal pregnancy, particularly human placental lactogen, glucagon and cortisol.

- Normal women show an approximate doubling of insulin production from the end of the first trimester to the third trimester.

- These physiological changes are likely to underlie the increased insulin requirements of established diabetics, and the development of abnormal glucose tolerance in gestational diabetics, in whom there is insufficient insulin secretion to compensate for the insulin resistance.

- The diagnosis of gestational diabetes mellitus (GDM) is arbitrary depending on where the 'cut-off' is placed on the normal spectrum of glucose tolerance in pregnancy.

- The renal tubular threshold for glucose falls during pregnancy. There is a tendency for glycosuria to increase as pregnancy advances and if all urine samples are tested, most pregnant women will have glycosuria at some time. Glycosuria is not a reliable diagnostic tool for impaired glucose tolerance or diabetes in pregnancy.

- In normal pregnancy, starvation results in early breakdown of triglyceride, resulting in the liberation of fatty acids and ketone bodies.

Pre-existing diabetes

Pre-existing diabetes (Fig. 5.1) may be divided into types I and II:

- Type I, insulin-dependent diabetes mellitus (IDDM) – juvenile-onset.
- Type II, non-insulin-dependent diabetes mellitus (NIDDM) – maturity-onset.

Incidence

In the UK, the prevalence of IDDM is about 0.5% and that of NIDDM about 2% (10% in Asian immigrants).

Clinical features

IDDM

- Patients usually present as children or young adults (age 11–14 years).
- IDDM most commonly affects Europeans who are not usually overweight.
- The clinical features relate to absolute insulin deficiency that, if untreated, causes thirst, polyuria, blurred vision, weight loss and ketoacidosis.

NIDDM

- Patients are usually older and often overweight.
- All racial groups are affected, but in the UK it is more common in Asian, Afro-Caribbean and Middle Eastern immigrants.
- NIDDM is caused by peripheral insulin resistance and a state in which the body is unable to compensate for this by increasing insulin secretion.

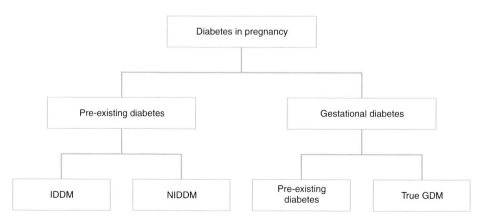

Figure 5.1 – Classification of diabetes in pregnancy.

- Individuals with NIDDM can have hyperglycaemia for a long period of time without clinical symptoms. It is therefore important to screen for possible occult long-term complications of the condition at the time of diagnosis.
- Although insulin is sometimes required to treat these patients, they do not become ketotic if it is withdrawn.

Diabetes (both IDDM and NIDDM) may present with the classical features mentioned earlier or with complications such as the following:

- *Candida* infection (pruritus vulvae)
- Staphylococcal skin infections
- Macrovascular arterial disease (coronary artery disease, cerebrovascular disease, peripheral vascular disease)
- Microvascular disease (diabetic retinopathy, diabetic nephropathy, diabetic neuropathy).

Diabetics have a reduced life expectancy related to accelerated arterial disease (two-fold risk of stroke, four-fold risk of myocardial infarction) and microangiopathy.

Pathogenesis

IDDM

This is an organ-specific autoimmune disease associated with serological evidence of autoimmune destruction of the pancreas and islet-cell antibodies. There is a genetic component and a strong association with the human leukocyte antigens HLA-DR3 and DR4. A possible viral component to the aetiology is thought to explain the seasonal incidence (spring and autumn).

NIDDM

There is no evidence of immune pathogenesis in contrast to IDDM. The genetic component is much stronger than in IDDM. The incidence increases with age and degree of obesity.

Diagnosis (in non-pregnant women)

Diagnosis of diabetes

If one of these criteria is met, it must be confirmed on a subsequent day by any of the three criteria below:

- Symptoms of diabetes plus plasma glucose ≥ 11.1 mmol/l (any time of day without regard to time since last meal).
- Fasting plasma glucose ≥ 7.0 mmol/l. Fasting is defined as no caloric intake for at least 8 hours.

- 2-hour plasma glucose ≥11.1 mmol/l during an oral glucose tolerance test (OGTT). The test should be performed using a 75 g glucose load dissolved in water.

Diagnosis of impaired glucose tolerance

During an OGTT, 2-hour plasma glucose ≥7.8 mmol/l, and <11.1 mmol/l performed as described above.

Pregnancy

Effect of pregnancy on diabetes

- Since normal pregnancy is associated with an increase in insulin production and insulin resistance, those women with IDDM and those with NIDDM (usually treated with insulin during pregnancy), require increasing doses of insulin as pregnancy progresses. Maximum requirements at term usually reach at least two-fold pre-pregnancy doses. Rapid increases in insulin requirements occur particularly between about 28 and 32 weeks' gestation, when the fetus is growing rapidly.
- Those women with diabetic nephropathy may experience deterioration during pregnancy in both renal function and particularly the degree of proteinuria. Deterioration in creatinine clearance is more likely in those with moderate and severe renal impairment (creatinine >125 μmol/l pre-pregnancy) and those with hypertension (see chapter 10). Any deterioration in those with mild renal impairment is usually reversed following delivery, and there is no long-term detrimental effect of pregnancy on renal function.
- There is a two-fold risk of progression of diabetic retinopathy during pregnancy and diabetics may develop retinopathy for the first time in pregnancy. The worsening retinopathy is often related to the rapid improvement in glycaemic control, which is a feature of early pregnancy, and to the increase in retinal blood flow. The risk is higher for those with IDDM than for those with NIDDM and is increased with bad metabolic control, diastolic hypertension, renal disease, anaemia, and severity of baseline retinopathy.
- Hypoglycaemia is more common in pregnancy (largely related to intensified diabetic control) and may be associated with relative 'hypoglycaemia unawareness'.
- For every 1% fall in HbA1$_C$, there is a 33% increase in hypoglycaemic attacks.
- Diabetic ketoacidosis is rare in pregnancy, probably in part related to the close supervision, but is a risk in the presence of hyperemesis, infection, tocolytic therapy or corticosteroid therapy.
- Women with autonomic neuropathy and gastric paresis often experience deterioration of their symptoms in pregnancy.

Effect of pre-existing diabetes on pregnancy

Maternal considerations

■ Women with poorly controlled diabetes have an increased risk of miscarriage.

■ Women with diabetes have an increased risk of pre-eclampsia. This risk is further increased if there is pre-existing hypertension or renal disease (the risk is about 30% if nephropathy and hypertension are present).

■ Pregnancies in diabetics with nephropathy are often complicated by severe oedema related to proteinuria and hypoalbuminaemia, and a normochromic normocytic anaemia that may only respond to treatment with recombinant erythropoietin.

■ Diabetes greatly increases the risk of infection during pregnancy, particularly urinary tract, respiratory, endometrial and wound infections. Vaginal candidiasis is very common in pregnant diabetics.

■ The caesarean section rate is increased to about 60%. This is at least partly related to early induction of labour.

Fetal considerations

■ There is an increased risk of congenital abnormalities. The level of risk is directly related to the degree of glycaemic control around the time of conception and directly correlated with the $HbA1_C$ (glycosylated haemoglobin). Women with $HbA1_C$ <8% have a risk of approximately 5%, but in those with levels >10%, the risk is as high as 25%. The risk is eliminated if normal $HbA1_C$ levels are achieved.

■ The specific congenital abnormality of diabetes is sacral agenesis, but this is very rare. Much more common are congenital heart defects and skeletal and neural tube defects.

■ The perinatal and neonatal mortality rates can be increased five- to 10-fold in babies of diabetic mothers but vary between centres. Mortality figures have fallen steadily over recent decades, largely related to improved diabetic control. If figures for congenital malformations are excluded, in some centres the perinatal mortality rate (PNMR) may be reduced to two-fold the non-diabetic population.

■ Fetuses of diabetic mothers are at risk of sudden unexplained intrauterine death (IUD). Again, this risk is related to the degree of diabetic control and is highest after 36 weeks' gestation. Various factors may explain these sudden losses including chronic hypoxia (more common in macrosomic babies, see later) in the presence of hyperglycaemia and lactic acidosis. It is not possible to predict IUD from the cardiotocograph (CTG), Doppler velocimetry or biophysical profiles.

■ Maternal hyperglycaemia, and particularly ketoacidosis, is detrimental to the fetus, and maternal ketoacidosis is associated with a high (20–50%) fetal mortality rate.

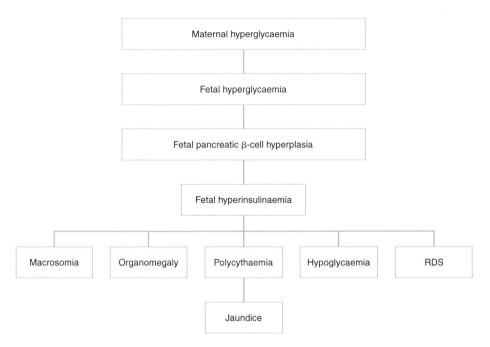

Figure 5.2 – Modified Pederson hypothesis. RDS: respiratory diabetes syndrome.

■ In contrast, maternal hypoglycaemia is well tolerated by the fetus.

■ Neonatal morbidity is increased in infants of diabetic mothers. The various complications may be explained by the modified Pederson hypothesis (Fig. 5.2).

■ Fetal hyperinsulinaemia may lead to chronic fetal hypoxia, which in turn stimulates extramedullary haemopoiesis, fetal polycythaemia and neonatal jaundice.

■ There is little evidence to support an increase in respiratory distress syndrome (RDS) in infants of diabetic mothers, although it is more common in babies of women with IDDM delivered by caesarean section. Obviously prematurity (more common in diabetic pregnancy) itself is associated with RDS.

■ Macrosomia has different definitions, but is conventionally defined as a birthweight >4.5 kg or >90th centile for gestational age. Insulin is an anabolic, growth-promoting hormone, and the macrosomic baby of the diabetic mother is characteristically fat and plethoric, with all organs, but particularly the liver, being enlarged.

■ Macrosomia is more common with poor diabetic control, but may also occur in cases of excellent control. The incidence of macrosomia increases significantly when mean maternal blood glucose concentrations are >7.2 mmol/l.

■ In the presence of fetal hyperinsulinaemia, when the cord is clamped, the neonate is 'cut-off' from its supply of glucose from the mother, and is at risk of neonatal hypoglycaemia.

■ Macrosomia is often associated with polyhydramnios (related to fetal polyuria), which carries the risk of premature rupture of the membranes and cord prolapse. Macrosomia increases the risk of traumatic delivery, particularly shoulder dystocia.

Management

■ Pregnant women with diabetes should be managed in joint pregnancy diabetic clinics by obstetricians and physicians with expertise in the care of such women. Such multidisciplinary clinics should be attended by specialist dieticians, nurses and midwives who are experienced in the care of pregnant women with diabetes.

■ There is evidence that outcomes can be improved with such tertiary level care.

Medical management

■ The most important goal of management is to achieve maternal near normoglycaemia as so many adverse perinatal outcomes are related to the degree of maternal diabetic control.

Table 5.1 – Complications of pregnancy in pre-existing diabetes

Maternal	Fetal
Increased insulin requirements	Congenital abnormalities
Hypoglycaemia	Increased neonatal mortality
Infection	Increased perinatal mortality
Ketoacidosis	Macrosomia
Deterioration in retinopathy	Late stillbirth
Increased proteinuria and oedema	Premature delivery (partly iatrogenic)
Miscarriage	Neonatal hypoglycaemia
Polyhydramnios	Polycythaemia
Shoulder dystocia	Jaundice
Pre-eclampsia	
Increased caesarean section rate	

- In order to achieve the desired level of control, pregnant women with diabetes will need to increase the frequency of home blood-glucose monitoring (HBGM), using glucose oxidase strips and preferably glucose meters.

- This is especially so in early pregnancy, when control is first tightened, and during periods when insulin doses are altered. HBGM also gives the woman the independence to adjust her own insulin dosages and this is to be encouraged.

- Target capillary blood glucose concentrations are <5.0–5.5 mmol/l fasting and <7.0–7.5 mmol/l postprandial.

- Outcomes such as birthweight correlate better with postprandial than with preprandial glucose levels. Neonatal hypoglycaemia and birthweight are reduced if the target for control in pregnancy is a postprandial level of <7.8 mmol/l compared to a fasting level of 3.3–5.9 mmol/l.

- Using postprandial targets also leads to better improvements in maternal $HbA1_C$ levels.

- Women with IDDM require increasing doses of insulin throughout pregnancy, and those with NIDDM usually require treatment with insulin during pregnancy, even if they are adequately controlled with diet with or without oral hypoglycaemic drugs outside pregnancy.

- Oral hypoglycaemic drugs (both sulphonylureas and biguanides) are usually avoided in pregnancy because they cross the placenta and there is a risk of this causing fetal hypoglycaemia.

- Women with NIDDM should be converted to insulin either before pregnancy or in early pregnancy. However outcomes are improved in women taking oral hypoglycaemic drugs compared to those in women who refuse insulin. Therefore their use may be justified in selected cases as the risks are outweighed by the risks of severe hyperglycaemia.

- Strict adherence to a low-sugar, low-fat, high-fibre diet is important in pregnancy, as this will aid glycaemic control. Starvation should be avoided because of the risk of ketoacidosis.

- The inevitable result of tighter control is an increased risk of hypoglycaemic attacks.

- For this reason, pregnant diabetic women will usually require a 'snack' mid-morning, mid-afternoon and before retiring at night. Relatives or partners may be taught how to administer i.m. glucagon injections to avert profound hypoglycaemia in situations where the pregnant, diabetic woman is unable or unwilling to eat or drink. The woman should be advised that glucagon provides only temporary relief from hypoglycaemia, and should always be followed by oral intake of glucose-containing food or drink.

- A four-times daily basal bolus regimen (nocturnal intermediate-acting insulin, such as insulatard, and three pre-meal injections of fast-acting insulin, such as human Actrapid®) allows maximal flexibility in altering the insulin dose to compensate for the increased requirements as pregnancy progresses.

■ Such basal bolus regimes also achieve better glycaemic control compared to b.d. mixed short- and intermediate-acting insulins (e.g. Mixtard®) and are associated with fewer instances of neonatal and maternal hypoglycaemia.

■ As in the non-pregnant diabetic, insulin should not be stopped during periods of intercurrent illness, and the dose may often need to be increased in the presence of infection.

■ Insulin requirements also increase with use of β-sympathomimetics and corticosteroids (see later).

■ Increasing numbers of women with IDDM are using the rapid-acting insulin analogues (Humalog® insulin lispro; Novorapid® insulin aspart) instead of conventional fast-acting preparations. Experience with these preparations in pregnancy is growing, and they seem safe and useful, especially in those with frequent and troublesome hypoglycaemia.

■ The degree of diabetic control may be assessed with $HbA1_C$ measurements.

■ Women should have a detailed ophthalmological examination in early pregnancy and periodically thereafter according to the severity of any retinopathy discovered. Laser photocoagulation can be used either to treat or prevent proliferative retinopathy in pregnancy.

■ Those women with diabetic nephropathy require regular monitoring of renal function (serum urea and creatinine, and creatinine clearance) and quantification of proteinuria (24-hour protein excretion) (see chapter 10).

■ Hypertension is found in 30% of women with diabetic nephropathy and up to 75% will develop hypertension by the end of pregnancy.

Obstetric management

■ An early dating and viability scan is recommended.

■ Because of the increased risk of congenital abnormalities, diabetic women should be offered nuchal translucency scanning and detailed ultrasound of the fetus at 18–20 weeks' gestation, including detailed assessment of the fetal heart.

■ Full hospital care is appropriate with regular blood pressure and urinalysis checks to detect pre-eclampsia.

■ Regular ultrasound assessment of fetal growth and liquor volume in the third trimester is advisable to detect or confirm macrosomia and polyhydramnios.

■ Particular care must be taken with the use of β-sympathomimetics (for premature labour) and corticosteroids (to induce fetal lung maturation) as these may lead to deterioration of diabetic control, hyperglycaemia and diabetic ketoacidosis.

■ Decisions regarding the timing and mode of delivery balance the risks of prematurity and its associated complications with the risks of late intrauterine death and macrosomia with its complications.

- Delivery before 38 weeks' gestation is rarely justified, especially in cases of well-controlled diabetes, a non-macrosomic fetus, and no evidence of pre-eclampsia.
- Most obstetricians plan delivery between 38–39 weeks, although in well-controlled diabetics, and in the absence of macrosomia or hypertension, the pregnancy may be allowed to progress to 40 weeks in the hope of spontaneous onset of labour.
- Pregnancies in women with pre-existing diabetes are not usually allowed to continue beyond 40 weeks.
- Overall, the risk of caesarean section (both elective and emergency) is increased in diabetic pregnancy, but although rates as high as 60% are common, this may be a realistic figure to avoid such devastating complications as shoulder dystocia.

Intrapartum management
- I.v. infusions of insulin and dextrose are administered throughout active labour and delivery via separate giving sets, to allow acceleration of glucose infusion and cessation of insulin in the event of hypoglycaemia.
- The capillary blood glucose should be estimated hourly, and the insulin infusion rate altered according to a sliding scale determined by the individual daily insulin requirements.
- The usual dose range is 2–6 units per hour. The target glucose level during labour and delivery is about 4–8 mmol/l, the aim being to avoid hypoglycaemia.
- The dextrose infusion (5% or 10%) should provide 500 ml of fluid every 8 hours.
- Following delivery of the placenta, the rate of infusion of insulin is halved.
- Postpartum, insulin requirements return rapidly to pre-pregnancy levels.
- Once women with IDDM are eating normally, s.c. insulin should be recommenced at either the pre-pregnancy dose, or at a 25% lower dose if the women intends to breast-feed. Most established diabetics are capable of adjusting their own insulin doses and can be advised that tight glycaemic control is not as important during the postpartum period.

Pre-pregnancy counselling

- This is one of the most important features of management of the diabetic woman in pregnancy.
- Women should be counselled that good control of diabetes and lower HbA1$_C$ levels lower the risk of congenital abnormalities in the fetus, and are associated with improved pregnancy outcome.
- Women should receive preconceptual folic acid (5 mg/day).
- The risk of diabetes in the child is 2–3% with maternal IDDM, and 4–5% if the father has IDDM.

- Pre-pregnancy counselling allows for optimisation of diabetic control prior to conception, as well as assessment of the presence and severity of complications such as hypertension, nephropathy and retinopathy.
- Thus a woman can be given a more accurate estimation of the level of risk of, for example, developing pre-eclampsia.
- If necessary, proliferative retinopathy may be treated with photocoagulation prior to conception.
- Contraindications to pregnancy include ischaemic heart disease, untreated proliferative retinopathy, severe gastroparesis, and severe renal impairment (creatinine >250 μmol/l.)
- Unplanned pregnancy is a risk factor for large-for-gestational-age infants in both pre-existing diabetes and GDM.

Pre-existing diabetes – points to remember

- The increased risk of congenital abnormalities is related to the degree of periconceptual diabetic control.
- Insulin requirements increase during pregnancy.
- Retinopathy may deteriorate during pregnancy.
- Diabetics, especially those with nephropathy and hypertension, have a greatly increased risk of pre-eclampsia.
- Neonatal and perinatal morbidity and mortality are increased in infants of diabetic mothers. Complications relate to the degree of maternal hyperglycaemia, fetal hyperinsulinaemia and macrosomia and may be decreased with tight diabetic control.
- Pregnant women with diabetes should be managed in joint pregnancy diabetic clinics by obstetricians and physicians with expertise in the care of such women.
- The most important goal of management is to achieve maternal near normoglycaemia.
- Outcome is improved if four-times-daily basal bolus regimes of insulin are used, and target blood glucose levels are based on postprandial capillary glucose estimations.

Gestational diabetes mellitus (GDM)

The definition of gestational diabetes from the National Diabetes Data Group (1985) is 'carbohydrate intolerance of variable severity with onset or first recognition during the present pregnancy'. Thus it includes women with pre-existing but previously unrecognised diabetes (Fig. 5.1).

Incidence

- This is hugely variable depending on the level of glucose intolerance used to define the condition (see later under 'Screening and diagnosis') and the ethnicity of the population under study.
- Using the definition for impaired glucose tolerance in the non-pregnant woman, the incidence is about 3–6%.
- In the UK, the prevalence is increased about 11-fold in women from the Indian subcontinent, eight-fold in South East Asian women, six-fold in Arab/Mediterranean women and three-fold in Afro-Caribbean women.
- The prevalence of GDM (with stricter criteria) in the UK is lowest (0.2–0.5%) in areas with a predominantly white European population and highest (1.5–3%) in inner city areas with a high proportion of ethnic minority women.

Clinical features

- GDM is usually asymptomatic and develops in the second or third trimester, induced by maternal changes in carbohydrate metabolism and decreased insulin sensitivity.
- GDM may be diagnosed by routine biochemical screening (see later) or may be suspected in the case of a macrosomic fetus, polyhydramnios, persistent heavy glycosuria or recurrent infections.
- Occasionally, GDM may be diagnosed retrospectively (with random plasma glucose or $HbA1_C$) following an intrauterine death or birth of a severely macrosomic infant.
- GDM is more commonly found in women with previous GDM, a family history of diabetes, previous large-for-gestational-age infants, obesity and older age at pregnancy.
- GDM is associated with increased perinatal morbidity (Fig. 5.2) and mortality in the same way, but to a much lesser degree, than pre-existing diabetes. These risks relate to macrosomia, which may develop as in the infant of the diabetic mother.
- Unlike pre-existing diabetes, there is no increase in the congenital abnormality rate, except in those women with unrecognised diabetes pre-dating the pregnancy and hyperglycaemia in the first trimester.
- GDM is associated with an increased risk of pre-eclampsia.

Importance of GDM

The importance of diagnosing GDM relates to three factors:

1. Women identified as having GDM have a greatly increased risk (40–60%) of developing NIDDM within 10–15 years.

- The diagnosis of NIDDM is often made late and 10–30% have established eye or renal disease by the time of diagnosis.
- It is possible that modification of diet and lifestyle with the correction or avoidance of obesity may prevent or delay the development of diabetes later in life. The relative risk of developing NIDDM almost doubles for each 4.5 kg gained.
- Even if prevention is not possible, earlier diagnosis resulting from careful follow-up (and counselling of the woman regarding the increased risk, and the advisability of regular (annual) blood glucose checks and the need to seek medical advice if she feels unwell) is beneficial and may prevent the development of microvascular complications.

2. A small proportion (1 in 1000) of women identified as having GDM will in fact have had diabetes pre-dating the pregnancy. They are therefore at risk from all the features associated with pre-existing diabetes in pregnancy, including in the case of IDDM, ketoacidosis.

3. Women with GDM have a higher incidence of macrosomia and adverse pregnancy outcome than control populations without GDM.
   - The relationship of postload glucose and fetal size exists throughout the spectrum of glucose tolerance and there is no threshold effect.
   - The controversy surrounding this issue relates almost entirely to the different diagnostic criteria used to define GDM. The more stringent the criteria, the more apparent the association.
   - The problems with clinical studies addressing pregnancy outcome in GDM are the lack of control of confounding variables such as maternal weight and age, and the lack of a 'control' or untreated group. Thus obese women and those with previous large babies are at risk of both GDM and macrosomic infants, and causality is difficult to establish.
   - Most cases of macrosomia are not associated with GDM and only 20–30% of infants of mothers with GDM have macrosomia.
   - Since it is possible to modify birthweight with treatment of GDM, most units do treat and therefore it is difficult to find data to address the issue of the effect of untreated GDM on pregnancy outcome.
   - Decreasing birthweight across a population raises issues regarding the relationship between low birthweight and adult hypertension and cardiovascular disease.
   - Diagnosing GDM and labelling of women as 'high risk' may itself adversely affect pregnancy outcome. The most obvious example is an increase in the caesarean section rate.

Screening and diagnosis

There is no consensus in the UK regarding who, when, how or indeed whether to screen for GDM.

Who?

- Some advocate universal biochemical screening.
- Some advocate screening for those >25 years of age.
- Many units still use 'clinical risk factor' screening, testing only women with:
  - Previous GDM
  - Family history of diabetes
  - Previous macrosomic baby
  - Previous unexplained stillbirth
  - Obesity
  - Glycosuria
  - Polyhydramnios
  - Large-for-gestational-age infant in current pregnancy.

When?

- The later in pregnancy the screen is performed, the higher the detection rate of GDM, since glucose tolerance deteriorates progressively with increasing gestation.
- The earlier in pregnancy the GDM is diagnosed, the greater the potential to treat hyperglycaemia and possibly improve outcome.

How?

- In the USA, a 50 g 'short glucose tolerance test' is used to screen all women at 26–28 weeks' gestation. This is then followed in screen-positive (1 hour level >7.8 mmol/l) women by a full 100 g oral glucose tolerance test (OGTT) for which there are specific criteria for the diagnosis of GDM.
- The World Health Organization proposed criteria equivalent to those for diagnosis of impaired glucose tolerance in the non-pregnant woman. Following a 75 g oral GTT, a woman is diagnosed as having GDM if either a fasting or 2-hour level is ≥7.8 mmol/l.
- Few dispute the need to diagnose and treat those with 'frank diabetes' (fasting ≥7.8 mmol/l or 2-hour level ≥11.1 mmol/l), but many units use higher 2-hour cut-offs than 7.8 mmol/l (for example 9.0 or 10.0 mmol/l) at which to diagnose GDM. The decision of individual units is likely to be influenced by resources and the ethnicity of the population.
- The Report of the pregnancy and neonatal care sub-group of the St Vincent Task Force on Diabetes Care in the UK recommended revision of the above (WHO) criteria to a fasting glucose of >6.0 mmol/l and a 2-hour post-load cut-off of 9.0 mmol/l.
- Some units favour screening and diagnosis using random or postprandial blood glucose measurements, since the oral GTT is unpleasant, unreliable

and irreproducible in pregnancy. Capillary or plasma blood glucose estimations are more easily repeated throughout pregnancy, but again there is no consensus concerning the ideal cut-off for diagnosis. This method does have the advantage of early and easy diagnosis of women with pre-existing but previously undiagnosed diabetes.

■ It is now widely believed that women with mild degrees of impaired glucose tolerance in pregnancy do not have a significantly worse perinatal outcome. Overly aggressive approaches to detection and treatment result in unnecessary intervention, maternal inconvenience, and more harm than may be prevented.

■ Several studies have shown that in women with impaired glucose tolerance (excluding frank diabetes) in pregnancy, intensive management with insulin and blood glucose monitoring confers no benefit compared to simple dietary advice and no monitoring.

■ The management of GDM is not controversial – only the degree of glucose intolerance that represents risk and therefore justifies management.

Management

As with pre-existing diabetes, close collaboration between obstetricians and physicians is essential.

Medical management

■ The mainstay of treatment is diet with reduced fat, increased fibre and regulation of carbohydrate intake. Carbohydrates with a low glycaemic index are advised. Obese women are given a reduced calorie diet, the aim being to maintain weight for the remainder of the pregnancy. Strict diets with limited calorie intake are not advised in pregnancy, because of the risk of ketonaemia.

■ It is often possible to identify certain elements of a woman's diet such as large quantities of high-calorie, carbonated drinks, fresh orange juice or high-calorie snack foods which, when removed, lead to rapid improvement in blood glucose levels.

■ As with pre-existing diabetes, HBGM is an integral part of management since it allows the woman immediate feedback.

■ Persistent postprandial hyperglycaemia (>7.5–8.0 mmol/l) or fasting hyperglycaemia (>5.5 mmol/l) despite compliance with diet, are indications for the introduction of insulin therapy. This should be in addition to, not instead of, dietary treatment. Women need to be reminded of the importance of dietary modification, although adherence to dietary advice is usually good during pregnancy.

■ Insulin is usually given as short-acting insulin before meals, although it may only be needed before some meals. In more severe cases, where there is fasting hyperglycaemia, intermediate-acting insulin may in addition be required at night.

- A four-times-daily basal bolus insulin regime, with adjustment according to postprandial rather than pre-meal glucose readings, gives improved glycaemic control and improved outcomes compared to b.d. mixed insulin and adjustment based on pre-meal glucose values.

- Despite the usual advice to avoid oral hypoglycaemic drugs in pregnancy, recent data suggest that newer sulphonylureic drugs (e.g. glibenclamide) that do not cross the placenta in appreciable quantities may be safely and effectively used as an alternative to insulin in GDM.

Obstetric management

- GDM is associated with an increased risk of pre-eclampsia and women should receive full hospital care with regular checks of blood pressure and urinalysis, especially towards term.

- Regular ultrasound assessment for fetal growth is advisable as this is likely to influence the timing and mode of delivery as well as possibly the decision to start insulin treatment.

- The risks to the fetus in cases of diagnosed and treated GDM are less than with pre-existing diabetes and therefore it is often not appropriate to advise routine delivery at 38 weeks' gestation, especially if GDM is well controlled.

- Routine induction of labour at 38 weeks' gestation and awaiting spontaneous labour by 41 weeks give equivalent rates of caesarean section and shoulder dystocia. Therefore each case should be assessed individually without blanket policies regarding timing of delivery.

Intrapartum management

- To minimise iatrogenic morbidity, the route of delivery should be based on the same maternal and fetal issues as in the non-diabetic woman.

- It is often possible to manage even insulin-treated women without insulin during delivery, especially those on small doses (<20 units/day) of insulin. This is because women do not eat much during labour. Those on larger doses of insulin are managed as women with pre-existing diabetes with i.v. dextrose and an insulin sliding scale.

- Following delivery of the placenta, the insulin infusion should be discontinued.

- For those on insulin and those in whom the diagnosis of GDM was made before 24 weeks of pregnancy, a formal 75 g OGTT 6 weeks following delivery is advisable to assess any degree of impaired glucose tolerance or diabetes present outside pregnancy.

- Women with GDM should be counselled regarding the risks of future diabetes (see p. 93) and be made aware of diabetic symptoms. They should receive lifestyle advice concerning exercise and diet, particularly reduced fat intake. Obese women should be encouraged to lose weight postpartum and all should be advised to avoid obesity.

Recurrence

- GDM usually recurs in subsequent pregnancies.
- Sometimes if a woman has lost a lot of weight between pregnancies and modified her diet substantially, she may not develop GDM.
- More often absence of GDM in a subsequent pregnancy relates to different diagnostic criteria.
- Women should be advised of the risk of recurrent GDM and future diabetes.
- Adequate contraception and planning pregnancies is important.
- Women with previous GDM should have fasting blood glucose checked prior to conception to detect diabetes that may have developed since the last pregnancy.
- In any case, they should have blood glucose checked in early pregnancy.

Gestational diabetes – points to remember

- The prevalence of GDM depends on ethnicity and the criteria used for diagnosis. Ethnic minorities are at increased risk.
- The importance of diagnosing GDM relates to the high risk of future diabetes, the detection of pre-existing diabetes, and a risk of macrosomia and adverse pregnancy outcome in severe cases.
- The GDM 'label' is not itself without risk; the risk of caesarean section is increased.
- Management of GDM is with diet in the first instance followed by insulin in resistant cases.
- Pregnancy and the puerperium provide a unique opportunity for education regarding lifestyle and dietary changes.

Further reading

Casson, I.F., Clarke, C.A., Howard, C.V. et al. (1997) Outcomes of pregnancy in insulin dependent diabetic women: results of a five year population cohort study. *Br. Med. J.*, **315**, 275–278.

de Veciana, M., Major, C.A., Morgan, M.A. et al. (1995) Postprandial versus preprandial blood glucose monitoring in women with gestational diabetes mellitus requiring insulin therapy. *N. Engl. J. Med.*, **333**, 1237–1241.

Dornhurst, A. (1994) Implications of gestational diabetes for the health of the mother. *Br. J. Obstet. Gynaecol.*, **101**, 286–290.

Garner, P. (1995) Type I diabetes mellitus and pregnancy. *Lancet*, **346**, 157–161.

Garner, P., Okun, N., Keely, E. et al. (1997) A randomised controlled trial of strict glycaemic control and tertiary level obstetric care versus routine obstetric care in the management of gestational diabetes: A pilot study. *Am. J. Obstet. Gynecol.*, **177**, 190–195.

Hawthorne, G., Robson, S., Ryall, E.A., Sen, D., Roberts, S.H. and Ward Platt, M.P. (1997) Prospective population based survey of outcome of pregnancy in diabetic women: results of the Northern Diabetic Pregnancy Audit. *Br. Med. J.*, **315**, 279–281.

Jarrett, R.J. (1993) Gestational diabetes: a non-entity? *Br. Med. J.*, **306**, 37–38.

Kjos, S.L. and Buchanan, T.A. (1999) Gestational diabetes mellitus. *N. Engl. J. Med.*, **341**, 1749–1756.

Report of the Expert Committee on the Diagnosis and Classification of Diabetes Mellitus. (1997) *Diabetes Care*, **7**, 1183–1197.

CHAPTER 6

Thyroid and parathyroid disease

Thyroid disease	Parathyroid disease
Physiological changes	Physiological changes
Hyperthyroidism	Hyperparathyroidism
Hypothyroidism	Hypoparathyroidism
Postpartum thyroiditis	
Thyroid nodules	

Thyroid disease

Physiological changes (see also Section B, Table 6)

- Hepatic synthesis of thyroid-binding globulin (TBG) is increased.

- Total levels of thyroxine (T4) and tri-iodothyronine (T3) are increased to compensate for this rise.

- Levels of free T4 are altered less by pregnancy, but do fall a little in the second and third trimesters (see Table of normal values, Appendix 2).

- Serum concentrations of thyroid-stimulating hormone (TSH) fall in the first trimester as concentrations of human chorionic gonadotrophin (hCG) (to which it is structurally similar) increase. hCG has thyrotropic (TSH-like) activity.

- TSH levels may also rise in early pregnancy.

- Hyperemesis gravidarum may be associated with a biochemical hyperthyroidism with high levels of free T4 and a suppressed TSH in up to 60% of cases.

- In the third trimester, TSH levels increase so the upper limit of the reference range is raised (7.0 μmol/l) compared with those in the non-pregnant woman (4.0 μmol/l). Similarly the normal ranges for free T4 and T3 are reduced (see Table of normal values, Appendix 2).

- Pregnancy is associated with a state of relative iodine deficiency that has two major causes:
  1. Maternal iodine requirements increase because of active transport to the fetoplacental unit.

2. Iodine excretion in the urine is increased two-fold because of increased glomerular filtration and decreased renal tubular reabsorption.

■ Because the plasma level of iodine falls, the thyroid gland increases its uptake from the blood three-fold.

■ If there is already dietary insufficiency of iodine, the thyroid gland hypertrophies in order to trap a sufficient amount of iodine.

■ Biochemical assessment of thyroid function in pregnancy should include assays of free T4 and, in some cases, free T3. Immunoradiometric assays of TSH are useful but should not be used in isolation because of the variable effects of gestation.

Hyperthyroidism

Incidence

■ Hyperthyroidism is more common in women than men (ratio 10:1).

■ Thyrotoxicosis complicates about 1 in 500 pregnancies.

■ 50% of affected women have a positive family history of autoimmune thyroid disease.

■ Most cases encountered in pregnancy have already been diagnosed and will already be on treatment.

Clinical features

■ Many of the typical features are common in normal pregnancy, including: heat intolerance, tachycardia, palpitations, palmar erythema, emotional lability, vomiting and goitre.

■ The most discriminatory features in pregnancy are weight loss, tremor, a persistent tachycardia, lid lag and exophthalmos. The latter feature indicates thyroid disease at some time rather than hyperthyroidism.

■ Thyroid-associated ophthalmopathy may occur before hyperthyroidism and is present in up to 50% of patients with Graves' disease.

■ If thyrotoxicosis occurs for the first time in pregnancy, it usually presents late in the first or early in the second trimester.

Pathogenesis

■ 95% of cases of hyperthyroidism in pregnancy are due to Graves' disease.

■ Graves' disease is an autoimmune disorder caused by TSH receptor-stimulating antibodies.

■ More rarely in women of child-bearing age, hyperthyroidism may be due to toxic multi-nodular goitre or toxic adenoma, or occasionally subacute thyroiditis, iodine, amiodarone or lithium therapy.

Diagnosis

■ This is made by finding a raised free T4 or free T3. Normal pregnant ranges for each trimester must be used (see Table of normal values, Appendix 2 and Section B, Table 6).

■ TSH is suppressed, although this may be a feature of early pregnancy.

■ Differentiation from hyperemesis gravidarum may be difficult (see chapter 12).

Pregnancy

Effect of pregnancy on thyrotoxicosis

■ Thyrotoxicosis often improves during pregnancy, especially in the second and third trimesters.

■ As with other autoimmune conditions, there is a state of relative immunosuppression in pregnancy and levels of TSH receptor-stimulating antibodies may fall with consequent improvement in Graves' disease and a lower requirement for antithyroid treatment.

■ Exacerbations may occur in the first trimester, possibly related to hCG production, and in the puerperium (especially if there has been improvement during pregnancy) related to a reversal of the fall in antibody levels seen during pregnancy.

■ Pregnancy has no effect on Graves' ophthalmopathy.

Effect of thyrotoxicosis on pregnancy

■ If thyrotoxicosis is severe and untreated, it is associated with inhibition of ovulation and infertility.

■ Those who do become pregnant and remain untreated have an increased rate of miscarriage, intrauterine growth restriction (IUGR), premature labour and perinatal mortality.

■ Poorly controlled thyrotoxicosis may lead to a thyroid crisis ('storm') in the mother and heart failure, particularly at the time of delivery.

■ For those with good control on antithyroid drugs or with previously treated Graves' disease in remission, the maternal and fetal outcome is usually good and unaffected by the thyrotoxicosis.

■ Rarely retrosternal extension of a goitre may cause tracheal obstruction. This is a particular problem if the patient needs to be intubated.

Management

Antithyroid drugs

■ Carbimazole and propylthiouracil (PTU) are the most commonly used antithyroid drugs in the UK. Most patients are treated for 12–18 months after the initial presentation of Graves' disease, but relapse rates are high, and some women are managed with long-term antithyroid drugs.

■ Both drugs cross the placenta, PTU less than carbimazole, and in high doses may cause fetal hypothyroidism and goitre. Neither is grossly teratogenic, although carbimazole occasionally causes a scalp defect – aplasia cutis.

■ The aim of treatment is to control the thyrotoxicosis as rapidly as possible and maintain optimal control of thyrotoxicosis with the lowest dose of antithyroid medication. The woman should be clinically euthyroid, with a free T4 at the upper end of the normal range.

■ Newly diagnosed thyrotoxicosis should be aggressively treated with high doses of carbimazole or PTU (45 mg or 450 mg daily, respectively) for 4–6 weeks, after which time gradual reduction in the dose is usually possible. A drug rash or urticaria occurs in 1–5% of patients on antithyroid drugs and should prompt a switch to a different preparation.

■ Women should be seen monthly in the case of newly diagnosed hyperthyroidism, but thyroid function tests (TFTs) are required less frequently in women stable on antithyroid drugs.

■ PTU is preferable for newly diagnosed cases in pregnancy (less transfer across the placenta and to breast milk), but women already on maintenance carbimazole prior to pregnancy need not be switched to PTU in pregnancy.

■ Doses of PTU at or below 150 mg/day and carbimazole 15 mg/day are unlikely to cause problems in the fetus.

■ Very little PTU is excreted in breast milk; only 0.07% of the dose taken by the breast-feeding mother is consumed by the breast-fed baby. It is therefore safe for mothers to breast-feed while taking doses of PTU at or below 150 mg/day and carbimazole 15 mg/day (0.5% of the dose is received by the breast-fed baby).

■ Thyroid function should be checked in umbilical cord blood and at regular intervals in the neonate if the mother is breast-feeding and taking high doses of antithyroid drugs.

■ There is no place for 'block-and-replace' regimens in the management of thyrotoxicosis in pregnancy. The high doses of antithyroid drugs required may render the fetus hypothyroid, and the thyroxine 'replacement' does not cross the placenta in sufficiently high doses to protect the fetus.

β-blockers

■ These are often used in the early management of thyrotoxicosis, or during relapse to improve sympathetic symptoms of tachycardia, sweating and tremor.

■ They are discontinued once there is clinical improvement, usually evident within 3 weeks.

■ Doses of propranolol of 40 mg t.d.s. for such short periods of time are not harmful to the fetus.

Surgery

■ Thyroidectomy is rarely indicated in pregnancy, but if required, may be safely performed in the second trimester.

■ It is usually reserved for those with dysphagia or stridor related to a large goitre, those with confirmed or suspected carcinoma, and those who have allergies to both antithyroid drugs.

■ 25–50% of patients will become hypothyroid following thyroid surgery, and therefore close follow up is required to ensure rapid diagnosis and treatment with replacement therapy.

Radioactive iodine

■ Radioiodine therapy is contraindicated in pregnancy and breast-feeding since it is taken up by the fetal thyroid (after 10–12 weeks) with resulting thyroid ablation and hypothyroidism.

■ Diagnostic radioiodine scans (as opposed to treatment) are also contraindicated in pregnancy but may be performed if a mother is breast-feeding, although mothers should stop breast-feeding for 24 hours after the procedure.

■ Pregnancy should be avoided for at least 4 months after treatment with radioiodine in view of the theoretical risk of chromosomal damage and genetic abnormalites.

Neonatal/fetal thyrotoxicosis

■ This results from transplacental passage of thyroid-stimulating antibodies (TSIs).

■ It occurs in 1–10% of babies of mothers with a past or current history of Graves' disease, but is most common in those with active disease in the third trimester, especially if poorly controlled.

■ It is possible to predict babies at risk by measuring the level of TSI, although the assay is not universally available.

■ TSH binding inhibiting Ig (TBI) levels >30 are predictive and >70 are strongly predictive.

■ It is important not to forget the possibility of neonatal/fetal thyrotoxicosis in babies of mothers with previously treated Graves' disease. A particular caveat is the woman on thyroxine (and therefore classified as 'hypothyroid') following previous thyroidectomy or radioiodine.

Clinical features

■ If the condition develops *in utero*, it may present with fetal tachycardia, IUGR or goitre. Without treatment, the mortality rate may reach 50%.

■ In the neonate, the condition may be delayed for 1 day to 1 week while maternal antithyroid drugs and/or blocking antibodies are cleared. Features include: weight loss, tachycardia, irritability, jitteriness, poor feeding, goitre, and in severe untreated cases, congestive cardiac failure. Without treatment, the mortality rate is about 15%.

Diagnosis

■ Serial ultrasound to check fetal growth, heart rate and fetal neck (for goitre) is advisable, especially in those mothers with poorly controlled or newly diagnosed thyrotoxicosis, when TSI levels may be high.

■ Percutaneous fetal blood sampling for measurement of fetal thyroid function is accurate, but carries an inherent risk.

Management

■ Treatment is with antithyroid drugs. In the case of fetal thyrotoxicosis, these are given to the mother. If the woman is euthyroid, these are combined with replacement thyroxine.

■ In the neonate, treatment must begin promptly, but is only needed for a few weeks, after which time maternal TSIs disappear from the circulation.

Hyperthyroidism – points to remember

■ Untreated thyrotoxicosis is dangerous for both the mother and her fetus.

■ Graves' disease often improves during pregnancy, but may flare postpartum.

■ Both carbimazole and propylthiouracil cross the placenta, and in high doses may cause fetal hypothyroidism and goitre.

■ The lowest possible maintenance dose of antithyroid drug should be used.

■ For those with good control of thyrotoxicosis on doses of carbimazole <15 mg/day or PTU <150 mg/day, the maternal and fetal outcome is usually good and unaffected by the thyrotoxicosis.

■ Women may safely breast-feed on these doses of antithyroid drugs.

■ β-blockers are safe to use short term if required for control of thyrotoxic symptoms.

■ Neonatal or fetal thyrotoxicosis, due to transplacental passage of thyroid-stimulating antibodies is rare, but dangerous.

Hypothyroidism

Incidence

■ Hypothyroidism is much more common in women than men.

■ It is especially common in those with a positive family history of hypothyroidism.

■ The condition is present in about 1% of pregnancies.

■ Most cases encountered in pregnancy have already been diagnosed and will be on replacement therapy.

Clinical features

■ As with hyperthyroidism, many of the typical features are common in normal pregnancy.

■ These include weight gain, lethargy and tiredness, hair loss, dry skin, constipation, carpal tunnel syndrome, fluid retention and goitre.

■ The most discriminatory features in pregnancy are cold intolerance, slow pulse rate and delayed relaxation of the tendon (particularly the ankle) reflexes.

■ Hypothyroidism is associated with other autoimmune diseases, for example pernicious anaemia, vitiligo and type I diabetes mellitus.

Pathogenesis

■ Most cases are due to autoimmune destruction of the thyroid gland associated with microsomal autoantibodies.

■ There are two principal subtypes: atrophic thyroiditis and Hashimoto's thyroiditis. The latter is the name given to the combination of autoimmune thyroiditis and goitre.

■ Hypothyroidism may be iatrogenic following radioiodine therapy, thyroidectomy or related to drugs (amiodarone, lithium, iodine or antithyroid drugs). Transient hypothyroidism may be found in subacute (de Quervain's) thyroiditis and in postpartum thyroiditis (see later).

■ The commonest causes encountered in pregnancy are Hashimoto's thyroiditis and treated Graves' disease.

Diagnosis

■ Diagnosis is made in finding a low level of free T4. Normal pregnant ranges for each trimester must be used, since the normal range for free T4 falls in the second and third trimesters (see Table of normal values, Appendix 2).

■ The TSH is raised, although this may be a feature of normal late pregnancy, or occasionally early pregnancy (see Section B, Table 6).

- The finding of thyroid autoantibodies may help confirm the diagnosis, but these are present in 10–20% of the population and should not be used in isolation.

Pregnancy

Effect of pregnancy on hypothyroidism
- Pregnancy itself probably has no effect on hypothyroidism.
- Although some believe that in later pregnancy an increased dose of T4 compared to early pregnancy and the non-pregnant state is required because of the weight gain in pregnancy, this is disputed.
- Earlier studies suggesting a need to increase the dose may have been based on increased TSH levels without making allowance for the physiological increase in TSH in the third trimester.
- If the dose does need to be increased in pregnancy, this is usually because of inadequate replacement prior to pregnancy.

Effect of hypothyroidism on pregnancy
- If hypothyroidism is severe and untreated, it is associated with inhibition of ovulation and infertility. Patients may complain of oligomenorrhoea or menorrhagia.
- Those who do become pregnant and remain untreated have an increased rate of miscarriage, anaemia, fetal loss, pre-eclampsia and low birthweight infants.
- The fetus is dependent on maternal thyroid hormone until autonomous fetal thyroid function begins at around 12 weeks' gestation.
- There is an association between untreated or subclinical hypothyroidism in the mother (as judged by raised TSH levels or reduced free T4) and reduced intelligent quotient and neurodevelopmental delay in the offspring. It is only maternal iodine deficiency that relates to severe permanent brain damage (neurological cretinism) in the child.
- For those women on adequate replacement therapy and who are euthyroid at the beginning of pregnancy, the maternal and fetal outcome is usually good and unaffected by the hypothyroidism.

Management

- Only very small amounts of thyroxine cross the placenta and the fetus is not at risk of thyrotoxicosis from maternal thyroxine replacement therapy.
- Most hypothyroid women are on maintenance doses of thyroxine of 100–150 μg/day, although the dose required varies between individuals.
- Provided a woman is euthyroid at the beginning of pregnancy, she will not usually require any adjustment to her thyroxine dose during pregnancy or in the puerperium.

- Thyroid function should be checked in all hypothyroid women, ideally pre-conceptually, or at least during the first trimester, to ensure adequate replacement.

- An isolated raised TSH in the first trimester is common and thyroxine doses do not need to be increased unless under-replacement is confirmed with a low free T4.

- It is not uncommon to find women who are under-replaced at the beginning of pregnancy, but any increase in dosage requirement is likely to be sustained postpartum, confirming a pre-existing undertreatment rather than an increased demand related to pregnancy itself.

- For those with newly diagnosed hypothyroidism in pregnancy, replacement with thyroxine should begin immediately. Provided there is no history of heart disease, an appropriate starting dose is 100 μg/day.

- In women on adequate replacement, thyroid function should be checked once in each trimester. Following any adjustment in thyroxine dose, thyroid function should be checked after 4–6 weeks.

Neonatal/fetal hypothyroidism

- This is very rare (1 in 180 000), and thought to be due to the transplacental passage of TSH receptor-blocking antibodies.

- These antibodies are more common in women with atrophic, rather than Hashimoto's, thyroiditis.

- The diagnosis may be suspected in the presence of fetal goitre.

Hypothyroidism – points to remember

- Untreated hypothyroidism is associated with infertility, an increased rate of miscarriage, and fetal loss.
- Pregnancy itself probably has no effect on hypothyroidism.
- For those on adequate replacement therapy, maternal and fetal outcome is usually good and unaffected by the hypothyroidism.
- Very little thyroxine crosses the placenta and the fetus is not at risk of thyrotoxicosis from maternal thyroxine replacement therapy.
- Provided a woman is euthyroid at the beginning of pregnancy, she will not usually require any adjustment to her thyroxine dose during pregnancy or in the puerperium.
- Neonatal hypothyroidism may rarely result from transplacental passage of TSH receptor-blocking antibodies, which are more common in women with atrophic rather than Hashimoto's thyroiditis.

Postpartum thyroiditis

Incidence

- The incidence is variable depending on whether active steps are taken to diagnose the condition, as well as local dietary intake of iodine.
- Estimates of incidence vary from 5–11%.
- It is more common in women with a family history of hypothyroidism and those with thyroid peroxidase (antimicrosomal) antibodies, in whom 50–70% will develop postpartum thyroiditis.

Clinical features

- Many cases are asymptomatic. Presentation is usually between 3 and 4 months postpartum.
- Postpartum thyroiditis can be monophasic, producing transient hypo- (40%), or hyperthyroidism (40%), or biphasic (20%) producing first hyperthyroidism and then more prolonged hypothyroidism (4–8 months postpartum).
- Symptoms are often vague and attributed to the postpartum state.
- In the hyperthyroid phase, there may be fatigue or palpitations.
- In the hypothyroid phase, there may be lethargy, tiredness or depression.
- Goitre (small and painless) is present in about 50% of patients.
- About 25% of patients have a first-degree relative with autoimmune thyroid disease.

Pathogenesis

- There is a destructive autoimmune thyroiditis causing first release of pre-formed thyroxine from the thyroid (rather than hyperfunction of the gland) and then hypothyroidism as the thyroid reserve is depleted.
- Fine-needle biopsy shows a lymphocytic thyroiditis (similar to Hashimoto's thyroiditis).
- It is possible that postpartum thyroiditis represents an activation of a previously subclinical thyroiditis caused by rebound in levels of antimicrosomal antibodies as the immunosuppressive effects of pregnancy are reversed.

Diagnosis

- Since up to 70% of women who are thyroid peroxidase antibody positive develop postpartum thyroiditis, some advise routine TFTs in such women at 2–3 months postpartum. Others argue that as many cases are asymptomatic and most resolve spontaneously, there is little value in screening.

- Postpartum thyroiditis is also more common in women with type I diabetes in whom screening may be justified.
- The diagnosis is often overlooked since the symptoms are vague and difficult to distinguish from the normal postpartum state.
- The diagnosis is made by biochemical testing to confirm hyper- or hypothyroidism.
- 80–85% of patients have positive antithyroid antibodies.
- To distinguish postpartum thyroiditis from a postpartum flare of Graves' disease, a radioactive iodine or technetium scan can be performed. This will show a low (as opposed to a high, as in Graves') uptake in the thyroid. Thyroid-stimulating antibodies will be absent in postpartum thyroiditis but present in Graves' disease.
- Distinction from Graves' disease is important, as Graves' requires treatment with antithyroid drugs (see later).

Management

- Most patients recover spontaneously without requiring treatment.
- The need for treatment should be determined by symptoms rather than biochemical abnormality.
- If treatment of the hyperthyroid phase is required, this should be with β-blockers rather than with antithyroid drugs. Antithyroid drugs reduce thyroxine synthesis and the problem in postpartum thyroiditis is increased release, not synthesis.
- The hypothyroid phase is more likely to require treatment. This should be with thyroxine replacement.
- Thyroxine should be withdrawn after 6–8 months to ascertain whether the patient has recovered spontaneously.

Recurrence/prognosis

- Only 3–4% of women remain permanently hypothyroid.
- 10–25% of women will suffer a recurrence in future pregnancies.
- 20–30% of women with thyroid peroxidase antibody-positive postpartum thyroiditis develop permanent hypothyroidism within 4 years. Therefore, long-term follow up of such women with annual measurement of TFTs is advisable.
- Postpartum depression is more common in thyroid antibody-positive women, irrespective of thyroid status.

> ## *Postpartum thyroiditis – points to remember*
>
> ■ More common in women with a family history of hypothyroidism, those with thyroid peroxidase antibodies, and IDDM.
>
> ■ Presentation is usually between 3 and 4 months postpartum.
>
> ■ May present with symptoms of hyper- or hypothyroidism but a high index of suspicion is needed.
>
> ■ The condition is caused by a destructive autoimmune lymphocytic thyroiditis.
>
> ■ Most patients recover spontaneously and treatment is not always required.
>
> ■ Postpartum thyroiditis is a significant predictor of future hypothyroidism.

Thyroid nodules

Incidence

■ Thyroid nodules are present in about 1% of women of reproductive age.

■ Up to 40% of nodules discovered in pregnancy may be malignant.

Clinical features

■ Features indicating malignancy are:
  - Previous history of radiation to the neck or chest in childhood
  - Fixation of the lump
  - Rapid growth of a painless nodule
  - Lymphadenopathy
  - Voice change
  - Horner's syndrome.

■ Features indicating de Quervain's (subacute) thyroiditis are:
  - Clear history of sore throat and systemic upset consistent with a viral infection preceding appearance of the nodule
  - Tenderness of nodule or goitre.

■ Very sudden onset of a nodule may suggest bleeding into a cystic lesion.

Diagnosis

■ Thyroid function tests and thyroid antibodies should be performed to exclude a toxic nodule or Hashimoto's thyroiditis.

■ A raised thyroglobulin titre (>100 µg/l) is suggestive of malignancy.

- Ultrasound is useful to distinguish cystic from solid lesions. The former are more likely to be benign, especially if <4 cm in diameter.
- Cystic lesions can be aspirated and the fluid sent for cytology.
- Fine-needle aspiration or biopsy of solid lesions should be considered, especially if there are other features of malignancy (for example, if rapidly enlarging or >2 cm; see earlier).
- Radioactive iodine scans are contraindicated in pregnancy.

Management

- If the lesion is malignant, surgery can be performed during the second and third trimesters, unless the diagnosis is made near term, in which case surgery can be postponed.
- Thyroxine should be given postoperatively in sufficient doses to suppress TSH, since any residual tumour is usually TSH dependent.
- If radioactive iodine is required for residual tumour or metastases, this should be delayed until after delivery.
- There is no adverse effect of pregnancy on the course of previously diagnosed and treated thyroid malignancies.
- In those with previously diagnosed and treated thyroid cancer, the diagnosis is usually papillary carcinoma, which affects younger patients. Thyroxine doses should be titrated to ensure the TSH remains suppressed throughout pregnancy.

Thyroid nodules – points to remember

- The possibility that a solitary thyroid nodule discovered in pregnancy is malignant must be considered.
- Malignancy is more likely with larger, fixed lesions, which are solid on ultrasound.
- Thyroid function tests should be performed to exclude other causes of nodules and goitre.
- Surgery may be performed during the second and third trimesters.

Parathyroid disease

Physiological changes

- Pregnancy and lactation are associated with increased demands for calcium.
- There is an increase in urinary loss of calcium.

- Both of these factors necessitate a two-fold vitamin D-mediated increase in calcium absorption from the gut.
- Vitamin D levels rise during pregnancy.
- There is a fall in total calcium concentration and serum albumin.
- Free ionised calcium concentrations are unchanged.

Hyperparathyroidism

Incidence

- Primary hyperparathyroidism is the third commonest endocrine disorder after diabetes and thyroid disease, although it usually presents after the child-bearing years.
- The incidence in women of child-bearing age is about 8 in 100 000.
- It may be caused either by parathyroid adenomas or hyperplasia.

Clinical features

- Women may be asymptomatic.
- Symptoms include: fatigue, thirst, hyperemesis, constipation and depression, but may be attributed to normal pregnancy.
- Other features include renal calculi and pancreatitis.

Diagnosis

- This may be difficult in pregnancy as hypercalcaemia is masked by the increased demands of pregnancy. An apparently normal total serum calcium may be found to be raised when corrected for the low albumin of pregnancy.
- Parathyroid hormone (PTH) levels are increased.
- Ultrasound can sometimes detect parathyroid adenomas but isotope studies are contraindicated in pregnancy.
- Hyperplasia or adenomas may not be detected until surgical exploration of the neck.

Pregnancy

Effect of pregnancy on hyperparathyroidism
- Hypercalcaemia may be improved by pregnancy and the fetal demand for calcium.
- The risks to the mother are from acute pancreatitis and hypercalcaemic crisis, especially postpartum when the maternal transfer of calcium to the fetus stops abruptly.

Effect of hyperparathyroidism on pregnancy

■ There is an increased risk of miscarriage, intrauterine death and premature labour.

■ The risk to the neonate is from tetany and hypocalcaemia, caused by suppression of fetal PTH by high maternal calcium levels. Fetal calcitonin levels are high to encourage bone mineralisation. Many cases of maternal hyperparathyroidism are diagnosed retrospectively following an episode of tetany or convulsions in the neonate.

■ Acute neonatal hypocalcaemia usually presents at 5–14 days after birth but may be delayed by up to 1 month if the infant is breast-fed. There may be associated hypomagnesaemia.

Management

■ If diagnosed pre-pregnancy, the ideal treatment is surgery.

■ Mild asymptomatic hyperparathyroidism can be managed conservatively.

■ The mother should be advised to increase her intake of fluids during the pregnancy, and if necessary a low-calcium diet and oral phosphate can be used.

■ All mothers of infants presenting with late (>5 days after birth) hypocalcaemic tetany or seizures should have their serum calcium concentration checked.

Hypoparathyroidism

■ This may be caused by autoimmune disease but occurs much more commonly as a complication of thyroid surgery.

■ The incidence of hypoparathyroidism following thyroid surgery may exceed 3%.

Diagnosis

Diagnosis is made in finding low serum free calcium and PTH levels.

Pregnancy

Effect of pregnancy on hypoparathyroidism
Pregnancy increases the demand for vitamin D and therefore doses need to be increased to maintain normocalcaemia in pregnancy.

Effect of hypoparathyroidism on pregnancy

■ Untreated hypocalcaemia in the mother increases the risk of second-trimester miscarriage, fetal hypocalcaemia and secondary hyperparathyroidism, bone demineralisation and neonatal rickets.

▣ Maternal hypocalcaemia may also be first diagnosed because of neonatal hypocalcaemic seizures.

Management

▣ Normocalcaemia is maintained with vitamin D and oral calcium supplements.

▣ The dose of vitamin D required increases two- to three-fold in pregnancy.

▣ Maternal serum calcium and albumin should be measured approximately monthly.

▣ Vitamin D therapy is best given as alfacalcidol (1α-hydroxycholecalciferol) or calcitriol (1,25-dihydroxycholecalciferol), both of which have short half-lives, allowing titration of dose against maternal calcium levels.

▣ Excessive vitamin D treatment leads to maternal hypercalcaemia and possible overmineralisation of fetal bones.

▣ The dose of vitamin D must be decreased again after delivery.

Further reading

Beattie, G.C., Ravi, N.R., Lewis, M. et al. (2000) Rare presentation of maternal primary hyperparathyroidim. *Br. Med. J.*, **321**, 223–224.

Girling, J.C. (1996) Thyroid disease and pregnancy. *Br. J. Hosp. Med.*, **56**, 316–320.

Haddow, J.E., Palomaki, G.E., Allen, W.C. et al. (1999) Maternal thyroid deficiency during pregnancy and subsequent neuropsychological development in the child. *N. Engl. J. Med.*, **341**, 549–555.

Hall, R., Richards, C.J. and Lazarus, J.H. (1993) The thyroid and pregnancy. *Br. J. Obstet. Gynaecol.*, **100**, 512–515.

Kotarba, D.D., Garner, P. and Perkins, S.L. (1995) Changes in serum free thyroxine, free tri-iodothyronine and thyroid stimulating hormone reference intervals in normal term pregnant women. *J. Obstet. Gynaecol.*, **15**, 5–8.

Mestman, J.H., Goodwin, T.M. and Montoro, M.N. (1995) Thyroid disorders of pregnancy. *Endocrinol. Metab. Clin. North Am.*, **24**, 41–71.

Tan, G.H., Gharib, H., Goeller, J.R., Vanheerden, J.A. and Bahn, R.S. (1996) Management of thyroid nodules in pregnancy. *Arch. Intern. Med.*, **156**, 2317–2320.

Wing, D.A., Millar, L.K., Koonings, P.P., Montoro, M.N. and Mestman, J.H. (1994) A comparison of propylthiouracil versus methimazole in the treatment of hyperthyroidism in pregnancy. *Am. J. Obstet. Gynecol.*, **170**, 90–95.

CHAPTER 7

Pituitary and adrenal disease

Physiological changes

Pituitary disease	Adrenal disease
Hyperprolactinaemia	Conn's syndrome
Diabetes insipidus	Phaeochromocytomas
Acromegaly	Addison's disease
Hypopituitarism	Congenital adrenal hyperplasia
Cushing's syndrome	

Physiological changes

Pituitary

- The volume of the anterior pituitary increases progressively during pregnancy by up to 35%.
- Postpartum involution is slower if the woman breast-feeds.
- Prolactin levels increase up to 10-fold during pregnancy and return to normal by 2 weeks after delivery, unless the woman breast-feeds.
- Physiological increases in prolactin are thought to be mediated via increases in oestrogen and progesterone and are related to the initiation and maintenance of lactation.
- Levels of luteinising hormone (LH) and follicle-stimulating hormone (FSH) are suppressed by the high concentrations of oestrogen and progesterone, and are undetectable during pregnancy.
- Basal growth hormone (GH) levels are unchanged by pregnancy, but human placental lactogen (hPL), which closely resembles GH, and a specific placental GH are secreted by the placenta.
- Levels of antidiuretic hormone (ADH) are unchanged by pregnancy.
- The placenta secretes adrenocorticotrophic hormone (ACTH) and corticotrophin-releasing hormone (CRH), but pituitary levels of ACTH are unaltered by pregnancy.

Adrenal

- Hepatic synthesis of cortisol-binding globulin (CBG) is increased.
- Levels of both free and bound cortisol increase during pregnancy and levels of serum and urinary free cortisol increase three-fold by term.
- Normal pregnant women continue to exhibit diurnal variation in ACTH and cortisol levels.
- Suppression by exogenous corticosteroid administration (as in a low-dose dexamethasone test) is blunted.
- Levels of angiotensin II are increased two- to four-fold
- Plasma renin activity is also increased two- to three-fold.
- Plasma and urinary levels of aldosterone are increased three-fold in the first trimester and 10-fold by the third trimester.
- Levels of urinary catecholamines, metanephrines and vanillylmandelic acid (VMA) are unaffected by pregnancy, although they may be affected by stress and drugs, as in the non-pregnant patient.

Pituitary disease

Hyperprolactinaemia

Aetiology

- Causes of hyperprolactinaemia include:
  - Normal pregnancy
  - Pituitary adenomas (prolactinomas)
  - Hypothalamic and pituitary stalk lesions (leading to removal of dopaminergic suppression of prolactin secretion)
  - Empty-sella syndrome
  - Hypothyroidism (TSH stimulates lactotrophs)
  - Chronic renal failure.
- Prolactinomas are the most commonly encountered pituitary tumours in pregnancy.
- Prolactinomas are divided into 'macro' (>1 cm) and 'micro' (<1 cm) prolactinomas.

Clinical features

- Cases with prolactinomas may present with:
  - Infertility
  - Amenorrhoea
  - Gallactorrhoea
  - Frontal headache

- – Visual field defects
- – Diabetes insipidus.
- In pregnancy, only the last three symptoms are discriminatory.

Diagnosis

- Outside pregnancy, diagnosis is by finding a raised serum prolactin level. Prolactin levels in normal pregnancy are greatly raised and are therefore unhelpful in diagnosing prolactinomas.
- Other pituitary function tests should be performed (such as thyroid function tests) if a pituitary tumour is suspected.
- Formal visual field testing should be used to confirm any suggestive symptoms or abnormality of the visual fields to confrontation.
- Diagnosis in pregnancy must rely on findings of pituitary magnetic resonance imaging (MRI) or computerised tomography (CT).

Pregnancy

Effect of pregnancy on prolactinomas
- Since the pituitary enlarges during pregnancy, there is a small risk that prolactinomas will enlarge to cause clinical problems.
- This risk is higher for macroprolactinomas (15%) than for microprolactinomas (1.6%) and probably highest in the third trimester.
- The risk of tumour growth is reduced (to 4% for macroprolactinomas) if the tumour has been diagnosed and treated preconceptionally.

Effect of prolactinomas on pregnancy
- Many women have received treatment (usually with bromocriptine or cabergoline) prior to pregnancy. Some require treatment with these dopamine agonists to suppress prolactin levels, permitting restoration of oestrogen levels and fertility, and to allow conception.
- In the majority, these tumours do not lead to complications in pregnancy.
- There is no evidence for an increase in congenital abnormalities, miscarriage or adverse obstetric outcome.
- There is no reason why women with prolactinomas cannot, or should not, breast-feed.

Management

- Dopamine-receptor agonists (bromocriptine/cabergoline) are usually discontinued once pregnancy is confirmed.
- These drugs may be electively continued in cases of macroprolactinoma.

- Serial prolactin levels are unhelpful to monitor tumour growth or activity in pregnancy.

- Formal visual field testing is only necessary for symptomatic women or those with macroprolactinomas.

- Features suggesting tumour expansion are persistent severe headache, visual field defects or the development of diabetes insipidus (see later).

- Any suspicion, especially in the case of macroprolactinomas, necessitates further confirmation with CT or MRI.

- Dopamine-receptor agonists are safe for use in pregnancy and these should be reintroduced if there is concern regarding tumour expansion. Cabergoline has a more favourable side-effect profile than bromocriptine, in particular causing less nausea. They are also safe to take during breast-feeding, although they may suppress lactation.

- Rarely, pituitary surgery or radiotherapy may be used to treat prolactinomas, but this should be delayed until after delivery.

Prolactinomas – points to remember

- These are the commonest pituitary tumours encountered in pregnancy, but rarely cause problems.

- Do not measure the prolactin level during pregnancy, as it is invariably raised.

- The risk of tumour enlargement during pregnancy is increased with macroprolactinomas >1 cm.

- Visual fields should be measured regularly in those with macroprolactinomas.

- If tumour enlargement is suspected, CT or MRI of the pituitary is indicated.

- Dopamine-receptor agonists are safe for use in pregnancy and during breast-feeding; these should be reintroduced if there is concern regarding tumour expansion.

Diabetes insipidus (DI)

Incidence

This is approximately the same as in the non-pregnant population, i.e. 1 in 15 000.

Clinical features

- Excessive thirst and polyuria
- Affected women will drink throughout the night and pass large volumes of dilute urine
- Plasma osmolality is increased (except in psychogenic DI; see later).
- Presentation may be with seizures, which are said to be more common in transient DI (see later).

Pathogenesis

DI is caused by a relative deficiency of vasopressin (antidiuretic hormone [ADH]). There are four types:

- *Central* – due to deficient production of ADH from the posterior pituitary that may be idiopathic or caused by enlarging pituitary adenomas, craniopharyngiomas, skull trauma or postneurosurgery, or rarely Sheehan's syndrome.
- *Nephrogenic* – due to ADH resistance and most commonly associated with chronic renal disease.
- *Transient* – due to increased vasopressinase production by the placenta, or decreased vasopressinase breakdown by the liver. The latter form of DI is found in association with pre-eclampsia, Haemolysis, Elevated Liver enzymes and Low Platelets (HELLP) syndrome or acute fatty liver of pregnancy (AFLP) (see chapter 11), and regresses after delivery.
- *Psychogenic* – resulting from compulsive water drinking and consequent polyuria.

Diagnosis

- Other causes of polyuria such as diuretics, hypercalcaemia and hypokalaemia should be excluded.
- In the non-pregnant woman, diagnosis is conventionally with a fluid deprivation test, when the patient is not allowed to drink for 15–22 hours during which time serial weights, urine and plasma osmolalities are measured. Following dehydration and a loss of 3–5% of body weight, ADH is stimulated and urine concentration occurs in normal women and those with psychogenic DI.
- In pregnancy, such dehydration is potentially hazardous and diagnosis should be attempted first by admission of the patient for observation, documentation of polyuria, and paired plasma, and urine osmolality measurements. Urine output ranges from 4–15 l/day.
- Confirmation of a diagnosis of DI is straightforward if the plasma osmolality (>295 mOsm/kg) or serum sodium (>145 mmol/l) is inappropriately raised in the presence of polyuria and a low urine osmolality (<300 mOsm/kg). This excludes compulsive water drinking.

- A 'short' water deprivation test, for example overnight, may be all that is required to demonstrate an increasing urine osmolality (>700 mOsmol/kg should be considered normal) with normal plasma osmolality and thus exclude cranial and nephrogenic DI.
- Failure to concentrate the urine in response to a rising or abnormally high plasma osmolality (>300 mOsm/kg) is diagnostic of DI.
- Administration of DDAVP (synthetic analogue of vasopressin) 10–20 μg intranasally allows differentiation of cranial (where urine concentration follows) and nephrogenic DI (in those who remain polyuric).
- Those with central DI have low ADH levels, but those with nephrogenic DI have high levels.

Pregnancy

Effect of pregnancy on diabetes insipidus
- Pregnancy may unmask previously subclinical DI.
- In those with established DI, there is a tendency to deterioration during pregnancy (60%). This may be due to the following:
  – Increased glomerular filtration rate of pregnancy
  – Placental production of vasopressinase
  – Antagonism of vasopressin by prostaglandins.

Effect of diabetes insipidus on pregnancy
- Severe dehydration and electrolyte disturbance are risks in undiagnosed or untreated cases. Complications include maternal seizures and oligohydramnios.
- In treated cases there is no adverse effect on pregnancy outcome. Labour proceeds normally and there is no contraindication to breast-feeding.

Management

- A confirmed or suspected diagnosis of DI in pregnancy should prompt a search for pre-eclampsia and AFLP in particular.
- DDAVP is safe for use in pregnancy for diagnosis or treatment of DI.
- For cranial DI, DDAVP is administered intranasally 10–20 μg b.d. or t.d.s. Serum electrolytes and plasma osmolality should be checked regularly to ensure adequate treatment and to avoid overtreatment and water intoxication.
- For nephrogenic DI outside pregnancy, chlorpropamide, which increases renal responsiveness to endogenous ADH, is sometimes used. This should be avoided in pregnancy because of the risk of fetal hypoglycaemia.
- Carbamazepine is also used for nephrogenic DI and is safer to use in pregnancy (see chapter 9).

Diabetes insipidus – points to remember

- Established or subclinical DI may worsen in pregnancy.
- Extended fluid-deprivation tests should be avoided in pregnancy and close observation with paired urine and plasma osmolality measurements may be sufficient to exclude DI.
- DDAVP is safe for use in pregnancy for diagnosis or treatment of DI.
- Transient DI may occur in pregnancy and is often associated with pre-eclampsia, HELLP syndrome or AFLP.

Acromegaly

Incidence

This is rarely encountered in pregnancy (5 in 100 000).

Clinical features

- Many patients are infertile because growth hormone-secreting pituitary adenomas often co-secrete prolactin and may also cause stalk compression, leading to secondary hyperprolactinaemia.
- Overall, about 40% of women with acromegaly have associated hyperprolactinaemia.
- The main clinical features are those of growth hormone excess, of which altered facial appearance, macroglossia, large hands and feet may be the most obvious.
- Headaches and sweating are other common symptoms.
- There is an increased incidence of hypertension and impaired glucose tolerance.

Diagnosis

- This may be difficult in pregnancy, because although basal levels of GH do not change, GH assays may detect hPL and placental GH.
- Insulin growth factor-I (IGF-I) is increasingly used as a diagnostic tool outside pregnancy, but this increases in normal pregnancy and cannot therefore be used.

Pregnancy

Effect of pregnancy on acromegaly
- GH-secreting adenomas may expand during pregnancy, but this is less common than with prolactinomas.

■ As with prolactinomas, expansion may cause visual field defects.

Effect of acromegaly on pregnancy
■ GH does not cross the placenta or adversely affect the fetus.
■ The risk of gestational diabetes and macrosomia is increased.

Management

■ Treatment prior to pregnancy is the ideal and this is usually with surgery and/or radiotherapy.
■ Bromocriptine is not as effective in decreasing GH levels as decreasing prolactin levels, but does work in about 50% of cases.
■ Octreotide (somatostatin analogue) decreases GH secretion and is used increasingly in the management of acromegaly, but there are no data regarding the safety of this drug in pregnancy.

Hypopituitarism

This may be caused by the following:
■ Pituitary surgery
■ Radiotherapy
■ Pituitary or hypothalamic tumours.
■ Postpartum pituitary infarction (Sheehan's syndrome)
■ Lymphocytic hypophysitis.

Sheehan's syndrome

This usually presents postpartum following postpartum haemorrhage and may lead to partial or complete pituitary failure.

Clinical features
■ Failure of lactation
■ Persistent amenorrhoea
■ Loss of axillary and pubic hair
■ Hypothyroidism
■ Adrenocortical insufficiency – nausea, vomiting, hypoglycaemia, hypotension.

Pathogenesis
■ The anterior pituitary is particularly vulnerable to hypotension in pregnancy, probably as a result of its increased size.
■ Most cases (90%) of Sheehan's syndrome are preceded by an episode of postpartum haemorrhage associated with hypotension.

Lymphocytic hypophysitis

This is an uncommon autoimmune disorder most common in late pregnancy and the postpartum period. Incidence is increasing as refined radiological and surgical techniques have permitted more precise diagnosis of pituitary dysfunction.

Clinical features
It presents with features suggestive of an expanding pituitary tumour:

- Visual field defects
- Headache
- Hypothyroidism
- Adrenocortical insufficiency – nausea, vomiting, hypoglycaemia, hypotension
- Diabetes insipidus.

Pathogenesis
There is extensive infiltration of the anterior pituitary by chronic inflammatory cells, predominantly lymphocytes, causing pituitary expansion. Various degrees of oedema and fibrosis may be present but no adenoma. Antipituitary antibodies have been described and this condition is associated with autoimmune thyroiditis or adrenalitis in 20% of cases.

Diagnosis of hypopituitarism

- Investigation reveals reduced levels of T4, thyroid-stimulating hormone (TSH), cortisol, ACTH, FSH, LH and GH.
- Secretion of ACTH, GH and prolactin in response to hypoglycaemic stress (insulin stress test) is impaired.
- Any patient with hypopituitarism should undergo pituitary imaging with CT or MRI to exclude a pituitary tumour.
- In cases of lymphocytic hypophysitis, MRI shows symmetrical (in contrast to pituitary adenomas) enlargement of the pituitary, suprasellar extension with displacement of the optic chiasm, pituitary stalk enlargement (rather than deviation) and abnormal dural enhancement with gadolinium contrast.
- Definitive diagnosis of lymphocytic hypophysitis can only be made by histological examination of pituitary tissue.

Pregnancy

Effect of pregnancy on hypopituitarism
- Subsequent pregnancies after Sheehan's syndrome and lymphocytic hypophysitis have been reported.
- Pregnancy is also possible with other causes of hypopituitarism.

■ Conception may require gonadotrophin stimulation of ovulation, but once pregnancy has been achieved, the fetoplacental unit produces enough gonadotrophin, oestrogen and progesterone to sustain the pregnancy.

Effect of hypopituitarism on pregnancy

■ If the condition is diagnosed and treated with adequate hormone replacement therapy prior to pregnancy, then maternal and fetal outcome is normal.

■ Previously undiagnosed or poorly treated hypopituitarism is associated with an increased risk of miscarriage, stillbirth and maternal morbidity and mortality from hypotension and hypoglycaemia.

Management

■ The management of acute pituitary insufficiency includes i.v. fluids, dextrose and corticosteroids.

■ The need for replacement hormones is determined by pituitary function testing, but most patients require glucocorticoids and thyroxine.

■ Corticosteroids are a logical and reportedly successful treatment for lymphocytic hypophysitis, especially during pregnancy and if there is no visual disturbance. However many cases undergo surgery because of misdiagnosis of pituitary tumour. This results in new hypopituitarism or failure of existing dysfunction to improve.

■ Cases of Sheehan's syndrome and lymphocytic hypophysitis have resolved spontaneously.

■ Unlike Addison's disease (see later) mineralocorticoid replacement is not required, because aldosterone secretion is not ACTH dependent and is consequently not impaired.

■ During subsequent pregnancy, requirements for thyroxine do not alter, but additional parenteral corticosteroids may be required (see later under 'Addison's disease').

Cushing's syndrome

Incidence

This is very rare in pregnancy, with only about 50 cases reported worldwide, as most cases are associated with infertility.

Clinical features

These may easily be attributed to the pregnancy:

■ Excessive weight gain
■ Extensive purple striae

- Diabetes mellitus
- Hypertension
- Easy bruising
- Headache
- Hirsutism
- Acne
- Proximal myopathy (discriminating feature in pregnancy).

Pathogenesis

- Outside pregnancy, 80% of cases of Cushing's syndrome are due to pituitary adenomas (Cushing's disease).
- In pregnancy, <50% of cases are due to pituitary disease and most are caused by adrenal adenomas (44%) or adrenal carcinomas (12%).

Diagnosis

- Pregnancy-specific ranges for plasma and urinary cortisol must be used.
- Low ACTH, with an increased cortisol level that fails to suppress with a high-dose dexamethasone suppression test, is suggestive of an adrenal cause.
- Localisation is with ultrasound, CT or MRI of the adrenals, or CT or MRI of the pituitary.

Pregnancy

Effect of Cushing's syndrome on pregnancy
- There is an increased rate of fetal loss, prematurity and perinatal mortality. The adverse outcome is only partly explained by maternal diabetes and hypertension.
- The neonate is at risk from adrenal insufficiency.
- Maternal morbidity and mortality are increased and severe pre-eclampsia is common.
- Wound infection is common after caesarean section, due to poor tissue healing.

Management

- Surgery is the treatment of choice for both pituitary-dependent and adrenal Cushing's syndrome.
- The management of women with this disease has been undertaken successfully during pregnancy.

■ Experience with cyproheptadine, metyrapone and ketoconazole in pregnancy is very limited, and metyrapone has been associated with severe hypertension. Ketoconazole should be avoided in systemic mycoses.

Adrenal disease

Conn's syndrome

Hyperaldosteronism is found in 0.7% of non-pregnant patients with hypertension but very few cases of primary hyperaldosteronism have been reported in pregnancy. This is probably due to under-reporting.

Clinical features

■ Hypertension
■ Hypokalaemia (serum potassium <3.0 mmol/l).

Pathogenesis

Primary hyperaldosteronism may be due to the following:

■ Adrenal aldosterone-secreting adenoma
■ Adrenal carcinoma
■ Bilateral adrenal hyperplasia.

Diagnosis

This is suggested by finding of:

■ Low serum potassium
■ Suppressed renin activity (compared to normal pregnancy ranges)
■ High plasma aldosterone (compared to normal pregnancy ranges).

Management

■ Hypertension is controlled in the usual way with methyldopa, labetalol or nifedipine (see chapter 1), and hypokalaemia is treated with potassium supplementation or potassium-sparing diuretics.
■ Amiloride is safe to use in pregnancy and high doses (e.g. 20 mg) may be needed.
■ Spironolactone, which is used as a potassium-sparing diuretic in Conn's syndrome outside pregnancy, should be avoided as it may cause feminisation of a male fetus because it is an anti-androgen.
■ Surgery for adrenal adenomas can usually be safely deferred until after delivery.

Phaeochromocytomas

Incidence

- Phaeochromocytomas are found in 0.1% of non-pregnant patients with hypertension but are only rarely encountered (<200 reported cases) in pregnancy.
- It is important to consider the diagnosis since when undiagnosed, the maternal and fetal mortality rate is extremely high.

Clinical features

- Paroxysms of:
    - Hypertension (may be sustained or labile)
    - Palpitations
    - Anxiety
    - Sweating
    - Headache
    - Vomiting
    - Glucose intolerance.
- Hypertension in pregnancy is common, and therefore a high index of suspicion must be maintained to achieve an early diagnosis.
- Cases often mimic pre-eclampsia.
- Hypertensive pregnant women with associated unusual features such as excessive sweating, headache and palpitations should be screened.

Pathogenesis

- Phaeochromocytomas are tumours of the adrenal medulla, secreting excess catecholamines
- 10% are bilateral
- 10% are extra-adrenal
- 10% are malignant.

Diagnosis

- This does not differ from that in the non-pregnant woman and is made by finding raised 24-hour urinary VMAs or catecholamines.
- Non-specific assays may give false-positive results if the woman is taking methyldopa or labetalol and screening should ideally be performed before antihypertensive therapy is commenced.
- Once the diagnosis has been confirmed, CT, ultrasound and MRI offer the best methods of tumour localisation, although the latter two are preferable in pregnancy.
- MIBG (131I-meta-iodobenzylguanidine) is contraindicated in pregnancy.

Pregnancy

Effect of pregnancy on phaeochromocytomas

- Potentially fatal hypertensive crises may be precipitated by labour, vaginal or abdominal delivery, general anaesthesia or opiates.
- Attacks in pregnancy may occur whilst supine due to pressure of the gravid uterus on the tumour.

Effect of phaeochromocytomas on pregnancy

- There is a greatly increased maternal and fetal mortality rate, especially if as in up to 50% of cases, the diagnosis is not made antepartum.
- The maternal mortality rate is about 17% in undiagnosed cases.
- The fetal mortality rate is about 26% in undiagnosed cases and 15% in diagnosed cases.
- Mothers may die of arrhythmias, cerebrovascular accidents or pulmonary oedema.

Management

- Adequate α-blockade with phenoxybenzamine or prazocin to control hypertension followed by β-blockade, if required, to control tachycardia.
- Surgical removal is the only cure, and optimal timing of tumour resection depends on the gestation at which the diagnosis is made.
- In general, if pharmacological blockade has been achieved prior to 23 weeks' gestation, then resection is performed. If the pregnancy is more than 24 weeks' gestation, then surgery becomes more hazardous and should be delayed until fetal maturity, when caesarean section with concurrent or delayed tumour removal is undertaken.
- Expert anaesthetic care is essential and both fetal and maternal mortality rates have improved significantly since the advent of α-blockade, which should be given for at least 3 days prior to surgery.

Phaeochromocytomas – points to remember

- A rare but dangerous cause of hypertension in pregnancy.
- Women with hypertension associated with unusual features of palpitations, anxiety, sweating or headache should be screened.
- Adequate α-blockade for at least 3 days prior to surgery is essential.

Addison's disease

Incidence

Addison's disease is rarely encountered in pregnancy and most cases have been previously diagnosed.

Clinical features

There is adrenocortical failure, causing both glucocorticoid and mineralocorticoid deficiency. This leads to:

- Weight loss
- Vomiting
- Postural hypotension
- Lethargy
- Hyperpigmentation, particularly in the skin folds, in recent scars, and in the mouth.

Investigation reveals:

- Hyponatraemia
- Hyperkalaemia
- Raised blood urea
- Hypoglycaemia.

Pathogenesis

- Most cases in the UK are now due to autoimmune destruction of the adrenal glands caused by adrenal antibodies.
- Tuberculosis is the other main cause.
- The autoimmune form is more common in women (female preponderance 2.5:1) and may be associated in up to 40% of cases with other autoimmune conditions, such as pernicious anaemia, diabetes or thyrotoxicosis.

Diagnosis

- This is made by finding a low 9.00 a.m. cortisol level, a raised ACTH level and a loss of cortisol response to synthetic ACTH (Synacthen).
- When interpreting the results of cortisol measurements in pregnancy, it is important to remember that both the serum total and free cortisol levels are increased. An abnormally low cortisol level for pregnancy may therefore fall within the normal non-pregnant range.

Pregnancy

Effect of pregnancy on Addison's disease

- Pregnancy has no effect on Addison's disease, except possibly causing delay in diagnosis. This is because many of the clinical features may be masked by or attributed to the pregnancy.
- There are certain times during the pregnancy when women with Addison's disease may require increased doses of steroid replacement (see later).
- Unlike autoimmune thyroid disease, autoimmune adrenal disease is not more common in the puerperium, although patients with established Addison's disease may deteriorate in the puerperium (see later).

Effect of Addison's disease on pregnancy

- Prior to the advent of steroid therapy, Addison's disease was associated with a high maternal mortality rate.
- Provided Addison's disease is diagnosed and treated prior to pregnancy, there should be no adverse effect on the pregnancy.
- Adrenal antibodies do cross the placenta, but neonatal adrenal insufficiency secondary to maternal Addison's disease is rarely encountered in clinical practice.

Management

- In contrast to adrenal failure due to pituitary disease (see earlier), in Addison's disease there is a deficiency both of cortisol and aldosterone.
- Maintenance treatment with both hydrocortisone (25–30 mg/day in divided doses) and fludrocortisone (usually 0.1 mg/day) is required.
- Treatment in the acute situation may require i.v. saline.
- Maintenance steroids should be continued throughout pregnancy. The safety of steroids in pregnancy has been previously discussed (see under 'Asthma', chapter 4, p. 63).
- Pregnant patients need to increase their dose of corticosteroids or receive parenteral hydrocortisone if they develop hyperemesis, infection or undergo any stressful event (e.g. amniocentesis).
- Labour should be managed with parenteral hydrocortisone (100 mg, intramuscularly, 6-hourly), since women with Addison's disease are unable to mount an increased output of endogenous steroids from the adrenal gland that normally accompanies labour and delivery.
- Clinical well-being and blood pressure together provide a good index of the adequacy of steroid replacement.
- Following delivery, the physiological diuresis may cause profound hypotension in women with Addison's disease. This can be treated with i.v. saline, but

prevention is possible if the higher dose of steroids to cover labour is weaned gradually over a number of days rather than over 24 hours, as it would be in patients on maintenance steroids for asthma or arthritis.

Congenital adrenal hyperplasia (CAH)

Incidence

- Classic CAH is rare (1 in 14 000). The gene frequency is 1 in 200–400 and the disorder is autosomal recessive. Milder forms are more common.
- If a couple have one affected child, the risk of a subsequent child having the disorder is 1 in 4.

Clinical features

The main problems are as follows:

- Masculisation of a female fetus
- Salt-losing crisis in a male neonate due to mineralocorticoid deficiency
- Precocious puberty in a male
- Female adults with CAH are often infertile, and may have psycho-sexual problems related to anatomical problems following corrective surgery for virilisation of the genitalia.
- Polycystic ovaries, anovulation, hirsutism and acne may occur in association with adrenal androgen excess.
- Amenorrhoea is common, and delayed menarche and premature menopause have been reported.

Pathogenesis

- All forms are caused by deficiencies of adrenal enzymes used to synthesise glucocorticoids. There is therefore increased production of cortisol precursors and androgens.
- Of these cases, 90% are due to 21-hydroxylase deficiency causing both reduced cortisol and aldosterone production, and increased androgen synthesis. These individuals have both glucocorticoid and mineralocortcoid deficiency and the 'salt-losing' form of CAH.
- Deficiency of 11-β hydroxylase is found in 8–9% of patients with CAH. This leads to accumulation of deoxycortisol that has mineralocorticoid activity and therefore these women may be hypertensive.

Pregnancy

Effect of CAH on pregnancy

- Few cases of pregnancies in women with CAH have been reported.
- There is an increased risk of miscarriage (inadequate corpus luteum activity), pre-eclampsia and intrauterine growth restriction.
- Occasionally, caesarean section is required because of an android-shaped pelvis.

Management

Pregnancy in women with CAH

- Increased surveillance should be carried out because of the risk of pre-eclampsia.
- Steroid replacement therapy should be continued at the pre-pregnancy dose, and most women with 21-hydroxylase deficiency require no alteration in pregnancy.
- Adequacy of corticosteroid replacement is usually monitored with androgen levels.
- Free testosterone levels are reduced or unchanged in pregnancy.
- 17-hydroxyprogesterone and androstenedione levels are raised and therefore unreliable markers of androgen suppression in pregnancy.
- If androgen levels are elevated beyond normal pregnancy levels, doses of corticosteroid should be increased.
- Despite high maternal serum androgens, placental aromatase converts these to oestrogens thus protecting a female fetus from masculinisation.
- Mineralocorticoid dosage usually requires no change.
- Increased corticosteroids are needed to cover delivery and with intercurrent stress such as infection.

Pregnancy when the fetus is at risk of CAH

- This situation arises if a couple have had a previously affected child.
- One option is termination of the pregnancy if investigation suggests an affected female fetus.
- Alternatively, dexamethasone given to the mother will cross the placenta and suppress the fetal adrenal production, preventing masculinisation of a female fetus. This strategy is controversial.
- High doses of dexamethasone (1–1.5 mg/day) are needed.
- Treatment should be started preconceptually, or before week 5 of pregnancy, to optimise the chance of normalisation prior to differentiation of the genitalia. However, genetic diagnosis is not possible until 12 weeks' gestation (chorionic villus biopsy weeks 10–11 + a week to obtain the result) and

should be carried out only if a couple have had a previously affected child and each of their genetic mutations is known.

- Only one in eight fetuses (1 in 4 risk of homozygote and 1 in 2 risk of female fetus) may benefit from these high-dose steroids, and 7 in 8 will be treated unnecessarily for 6 weeks.

- If it is thought that a female fetus is affected, treatment of the mother should continue until term to prevent late masculinisation and neuroendocrine effects of exposure to high androgen levels.

- All female neonates should receive corticosteroids, both to treat CAH and because the neonatal adrenal glands will be suppressed following long-term, high-dose dexamethasone treatment of the mother.

- Male fetuses do not need to be treated *in utero.*

- Unfortunately, prevention of virilisation with the regimen mentioned earlier is not always successful and the parents must be fully counselled regarding the risks and benefits of use of such high doses of steroids throughout pregnancy.

Further reading

Pituitary disease

Beressi, N., Beressir, J-P., Cohen, R. and Modigliani, E. (1999) Lymphocytic hypophysitis. *Ann. Med. Intern.,* **150,** 327–334.

Hanson, R.S., Powrie, R.O. and Larson, L. (1997) Diabetes insipidus in pregnancy – A treatable cause of oligohydramnios. *Obstet. Gynecol.,* **89,** 816–817.

Montoro, M.N. and Mestman, J.H. (1994) Pituitary diseases in pregnancy. *Infert. Reprod. Med. Clin. North Am.,* **5,** 729–747.

Nasrat, H., Wali, F.N. and Warda, A. (1997) Diabetes insipidus, a rare complication of HELLP syndrome. Report of local experience and review of the literature. *J. Obstet. Gynaecol.,* **17,** 64–65.

Rossi, A-M., Vilska, S. and Heinonen, P.K. (1995) Outcome of pregnancies in women with treated or untreated hyperprolactinaemia. *Eur. J. Obstet. Gynaecol.,* **63,** 143–146.

Adrenal disease

Botchan, A., Hauser, R., Kupfermine, M. et al. (1995) Phaeochromocytoma in pregnancy. Case report and review of the literature. *Obstet. Gynecol. Surv.,* **50,** 321.

Garner, P.R. (1998) Congenital adrenal hyperplasia in pregnancy. *Semin. Perinatol.,* **22,** 446–456.

Harper, M.A., Murnaghan, G.A., Kennedy, L., Hadden, D.R. and Atkinson, A.B. (1989) Phaeochromocytoma in pregnancy. Five cases and a review of the literature. *Br. J. Obstet. Gynaecol.,* **96,** 594–606.

Khunda, S. (1972) Pregnancy and Addison's disease. *Obstet. Gynecol.,* **39,** 431–434.

CHAPTER 8

Connective-tissue disease

Rheumatoid arthritis	Antiphospholipid syndrome
Systemic lupus erythematosus	Scleroderma
Neonatal lupus syndromes	Ehlers–Danlos syndrome
Pregnancy-associated osteoporosis	

Rheumatoid arthritis

Incidence

- The adult form of the disease is more common in women (female to male ratio 3:1).
- Approximately 1 woman in every 1000–2000 pregnancies is affected.

Clinical features

- Rheumatoid arthritis is a chronic inflammatory disease affecting primarily the synovial joints.
- The prominent symptoms are joint pain and morning stiffness.
- Signs include swelling, warmth and tenderness with limitation of movement.
- There is symmetrical involvement, particularly of the metacarpophalangeal, proximal interphalangeal and wrist joints.
- Deformities such as ulnar deviation of the metacarpophalangeal joints and Swan neck and Boutonniere deformities of the fingers may be apparent in the later stages of the disease.
- Rheumatoid arthritis is a systemic disorder. Extra-articular features include: fatigue, vasculitis and subcutaneous (rheumatoid) nodules, haematological abnormalities, pulmonary granulomas and cardiac involvement.
- The eyes may be involved with scleritis, scleromalacia or most commonly (15%) Sjögren's syndrome (dry eyes and mouth).

Pathogenesis

- Rheumatoid arthritis is an autoimmune disorder involving autoantibodies directed against immunoglobulins.

- Immune complexes are common in the synovial fluid and circulation.
- The two main pathological characteristics are inflammation and proliferation of the synovium.
- There is progressive joint damage causing severe disability.
- There is an association with the human leukocyte antigen HLA-D4 (70%).

Diagnosis and immunology

- About 80–90% of patients are positive for rheumatoid factor (RhF).
- Antinuclear antibodies are positive in about 30% of cases.
- Anaemia (normochromic, normocytic) is related to the degree of disease activity.
- The erythrocyte sedimentation rate (ESR) and C-reactive protein (CRP) are also used as markers of disease activity, but the ESR is unreliable in pregnancy as it is normally elevated.
- Sjögren's syndrome is particularly associated with anti-Ro and anti-La antibodies (see later under 'Neonatal lupus syndromes') i.e. antibodies directed against extractable nuclear antigens (ENAs).
- About 5–10% of patients with rheumatoid arthritis have antiphospholipid antibodies (see later), but antiphospholipid syndrome is unusual (see later).

Pregnancy

Effect of pregnancy on rheumatoid arthritis

- Up to 75% of women with rheumatoid arthritis experience improvement during pregnancy, although only about 16% enter complete remission.
- Various theories have been proposed to explain the improvement including:
  - Raised cortisol levels
  - A maternal immune response to fetal paternally inherited HLA class II gene products
  - Decrease in T-cell-mediated immunity
  - High oestrogen levels
  - Pregnancy-specific proteins such as α2-glycoprotein (PAG) (in experimental models, PAG improves arthritis)
  - Removal of immune complexes by the placenta.
- Improvement usually begins during the first trimester and rheumatoid nodules may also disappear.
- Of those who experience remission, 90% suffer postpartum exacerbations. This may be related to resurgence of T-cell-mediated immunity in the puerperium.
- Postpartum flares are made worse by breast-feeding, possibly related to prolactin.

- There is an increase in the incidence of first presentation of rheumatoid arthritis in the postpartum period, particularly after the first pregnancy.

Effect of rheumatoid arthritis on pregnancy

- Unlike systemic lupus erythematosus (SLE), there seems to be no adverse affect of rheumatoid arthritis on pregnancy.
- Neither the fertility rate nor spontaneous abortion rate is significantly altered.
- Infants of women who have anti-Ro antibodies are at risk of neonatal lupus (see later).
- Atlanto-axial subluxation is a rare complication of a general anaesthetic for caesarean section, and very rarely, limitation of hip abduction is severe enough to impede vaginal delivery.
- The main concerns relate to the safety during pregnancy and lactation of the medications used to treat rheumatoid arthritis (see below).

Management

Simple analgesics

Paracetamol should be the first-line analgesic and there are no known adverse effects specific to pregnancy or the fetus.

Non-steroidal anti-inflammatory drugs

- Neither aspirin nor non-steroidal anti-inflammatory drugs (NSAIDs) are teratogenic.
- NSAIDs may cause infertility via 'luteinised unruptured follicle syndrome' or impairment of blastocyst implantation.
- Salicylates (in high doses) and NSAIDs may increase the risk of neonatal haemorrhage via inhibition of platelet function.
- NSAIDs may also lead to oligohydramnios via effects on the fetal kidney, and may cause premature closure of the ductus arteriosus because they are prostaglandin synthetase inhibitors. However, both constriction of the ductus arteriosus and impairment of fetal renal function are reversible after discontinuation of NSAIDs.
- The risk of premature closure of the ductus may have been exaggerated since this has not been encountered when indomethacin is used for the treatment of premature labour.
- NSAIDs are usually avoided, especially in the third trimester.
- In occasional circumstances, and especially prior to 28 weeks' gestation, NSAIDS may be used for control of arthritic pain if there are relative

contraindications to steroids (for example, in patients on heparin therapy) or if steroids are relatively ineffective (e.g. in ankylosing spondylitis).

■ If NSAIDs are used during pregnancy, they should be discontinued by 32–34 weeks' gestation.

■ The recently introduced cyclo-oxygenase type-2-selective (COX-2) NSAIDs, although currently contraindicated in pregnancy, have been reported to show only minor renal and no ductal effects on the fetus when used to prevent premature labour.

Corticosteroids

■ Corticosteroids may be continued during pregnancy and are preferable to NSAIDs if paracetamol is insufficient to control symptoms in the third trimester.

■ Women – and their doctors – are often reluctant to use corticosteroids, but this concern is misplaced.

■ For a discussion on safety of corticosteroids in pregnancy, see chapter 4 under 'Asthma', p. 63.

■ Pregnant women taking steroids are at increased risk of gestational diabetes and premature rupture of the membranes.

■ If a woman is on long-term maintenance steroids (>7.5 mg prednisolone for >2 weeks), parenteral steroids should be administered to cover the stress of labour and delivery, regardless of the route of delivery.

Azathioprine

■ Azathioprine is the commonest cytotoxic drug used for treatment of rheumatoid arthritis and SLE and is safe to use in pregnancy. This is partly because the fetal liver lacks the enzyme that converts azathioprine to its active metabolites.

■ There is a theoretical risk of azathioprine inducing chromosome aberrations in germ cells, which might lead to future malignancies or impairment of reproduction in female offspring. However, the offspring of renal transplant mothers and women with SLE treated with azathioprine appear normal at birth and in early childhood, although no data regarding fertility are available.

■ Low concentrations of azathioprine are found in breast milk, but the standard advice is for women requiring azathioprine to avoid breast-feeding. This is because of a theoretical risk of immunosuppression in the neonate. It could be argued that the benefits of breast-feeding outweigh this small theoretical risk.

Antimalarials

■ Antimalarial drugs such as hydroxychloroquine, used in rheumatoid arthritis and to prevent flares in SLE, are safe to use in doses used for malarial prophylaxis.

- There was concern that larger doses, used in the management of rheumatic disorders, could accumulate in the fetal uveal tract, resulting in retinopathy.
- Pregnancies in women exposed to chloroquine and hydroxychloroquine have congenital abnormality rates no higher than background rates in the general/unexposed population.
- There is increasing experience of hydroxychloroquine use in pregnant women with SLE and no adverse effect on the neonates has been demonstrated.
- Cessation of hydroxychloroquine therapy in early pregnancy is illogical for two reasons. Firstly it has a very long half-life such that the fetus remains exposed to the drug for several weeks following discontinuation of maternal therapy. Secondly, discontinuation of hydroxychloroquine is associated with a risk of lupus flare.

d-penicillamine

- d-penicillamine is a chelating agent used particularly in the management of the extra-articular features of rheumatoid arthritis.
- The drug crosses the placenta and in high doses may be a teratogen associated with abnormalities of connective tissue. The risk of congenital collagen defect is about 5% and therefore it should be stopped pre-conceptually in women with rheumatic diseases.
- However, about 90 reported cases of maternal penicillamine use suggest that it is relatively safe.
- The continued use of penicillamine is crucial for successful outcome of pregnancy in Wilson's disease.

Gold salts

- Although teratogenic in animals, there is no conclusive evidence for a teratogenic effect in humans.
- Gold salts should be avoided if possible during pregnancy and are rarely needed as rheumatoid arthritis usually improves.
- For women who are stable on gold therapy, the risk of a flare may outweigh any risk to the fetus from continuation of therapy.

Sulfasalazine

- Sulfasalazine is another second-line agent that has been used extensively in the treatment of inflammatory bowel disease in pregnancy.
- It is cleaved into 5-aminosalicylic acid and sulphapyridine in the colon.
- It may be safely continued throughout pregnancy, and breast-feeding.
- It is a dihydrofolate reductase inhibitor and therefore associated with an increased risk of neural tube defects, oral clefts and cardiovascular defects. Concomitant folate (5 mg/day) supplementation is recommended.

Cytotoxic drugs

- Cyclophosphamide, methotrexate and chlorambucil are all contraindicated in pregnancy.
- Cyclophosphamide and chlorambucil are alkylating agents. The risk of congenital defects in cyclophosphamide-exposed children is about 16–22%.
- Cyclophosphamide may be used later in pregnancy for life-threatening maternal disease.
- Methotrexate, a folic acid antagonist, is a powerful teratogen, and causes miscarriage or congenital abnormalities if administered in early pregnancy. It must be discontinued at least 3 months prior to conception.

Rheumatoid arthritis – points to remember

- Up to 75% of women with rheumatoid arthritis improve during pregnancy.
- Of those who experience remission, 90% suffer postpartum exacerbations.
- There are no adverse effects of rheumatoid arthritis on pregnancy outcome.
- Infants of woman who have anti-Ro antibodies are at risk of neonatal lupus.
- Atlanto-axial subluxation is a rare complication of a general anaesthetic for caesarean section.
- Limitation of hip abduction may be severe enough to impede vaginal delivery.
- If paracetamol-based analgesics are insufficient, corticosteroids should be used in preference to NSAIDs.
- Sulphasalazine, hydroxychloroquine and azathioprine can be safely continued in pregnancy.
- Cyclophosphamide, methotrexate and chlorambucil are all contraindicated in pregnancy.

Systemic lupus erythematosus (SLE)

Incidence

- Women are affected much more commonly than men (ratio 9:1), particularly during the child-bearing years (ratio 15:1).
- The incidence is approximately 1 in 1000 women and may be increasing.

Clinical features

- SLE is a systemic connective tissue disease characterised by periods of disease activity (flares) and remissions.
- The average age at diagnosis is about 30 years and about 6% of patients have other autoimmune disorders.
- SLE is heterogeneous with a variety of clinical and antibody patterns.
- Joint involvement is the commonest clinical feature (90%). Arthritis is non-erosive and peripheral.
- Other features include skin involvement (80%), for example malar rash, photosensitivity, vasculitic lesions on the fingertips and nail folds, Raynaud's phenomenon and discoid lupus.
- There may be serositis (pleuritis, pericarditis), renal involvement (particularly proteinuria) and neurological involvement (psychosis or chorea).
- Haematological manifestations include haemolytic anaemia, thrombocytopenia and lymphopenia or leukopenia.

Pathogenesis

- The cause of SLE is not known, but involves both a genetic predisposition and environmental triggers such as ultraviolet light or viral infection.
- There is polyclonal B-cell activation, impaired T-cell regulation of the immune response and failure to remove immune complexes.
- There are circulating non-organ-specific autoantibodies.
- Deposition of immune complexes causes vasculitis and glomerulonephritis.

Diagnosis

- Specific clinical and laboratory criteria (American Rheumatic Association) exist for the diagnosis of SLE, but many patients have a lupus-like illness without fulfilling these.
- A full blood count may show a normochromic normocytic anaemia, neutropenia and thrombocytopenia.
- The ESR is raised, the CRP is normal, and serum complement levels are reduced during active disease.
- The most common auto-antibody found in 96% of SLE patients is antinuclear antibody (ANA), but the most specific are antibodies to double-stranded DNA (found in 78% of patients).
- In addition, patients may have antibodies to extractable nuclear antigens (ENAs), for example anti-Ro and anti-La or to phospholipids, i.e. anticardiolipin antibodies.

- The anti-Ro (present in about 30%) and antiphospholipid antibodies (APA – present in about 30%) considered later are of particular relevance to pregnancy.

Pregnancy

Effect of pregnancy on SLE

- Pregnancy increases the likelihood of flare, from about 40% to about 60%.
- There is little evidence from recent studies to confirm the suspicion that flares are more likely immediately postpartum.
- Lupus flares, most commonly involving the skin and joints, may occur at any stage of pregnancy or the puerperium. It is not possible to predict when, or if, an individual patient will flare.
- Flares may be difficult to diagnose during pregnancy since many features such as hair loss, oedema, facial erythema, fatigue, anaemia, raised ESR and musculoskeletal pain also occur in normal pregnancy.
- Flares are not prevented with prophylactic steroids or routine increases of dose, and such prophylactic therapy is not recommended either ante- or postpartum.
- In women with lupus nephritis, pregnancy does not seem to jeopardise renal function in the long term, although SLE nephropathy may manifest for the first time in pregnancy. The risk of deterioration is greater the higher the baseline serum creatinine, although women with moderate renal impairment (serum creatinine >125 µmol/l) may have uncomplicated pregnancies.
- Women should be advised to delay pregnancy until at least 6 months after a lupus nephritis flare.

Effect of SLE on pregnancy

- The increased risks of spontaneous miscarriage, fetal death, pre-eclampsia, preterm delivery and intrauterine growth restriction (IUGR) seen in SLE pregnancies is related to the presence of anticardiolipin antibodies or lupus anticoagulant (APA), lupus nephritis or hypertension and active disease at the time of conception or first presentation of SLE during pregnancy.
- Pregnancy outcome is particularly affected by renal disease. Even quiescent renal lupus is associated with increased risk of fetal loss, pre-eclampsia and IUGR, particularly if there is hypertension or proteinuria.
- For women in remission, but without hypertension, renal involvement or APA, the risk of pregnancy loss and pre-eclampsia is probably no higher than in the general population.
- Chorea is a very rare complication of pregnancy in women with SLE or APA.

Management

■ Ideally this should begin with preconception counselling. Knowledge of the anti-Ro, antiphospholipid, renal and blood pressure status allows prediction of the risks to the woman and her fetus.

■ Outcome is improved if conception occurs during disease remission.

■ Pregnancy care is best undertaken by a multidisciplinary team in combined clinics, where physicians and obstetricians can regularly monitor disease activity as well as fetal growth parameters, uterine artery Doppler bloodflow examination at 20–24 weeks' gestation, and umbilical artery blood flow from 24 weeks' gestation.

■ Disease flares must be actively managed. Corticosteroids are the drugs of choice.

■ The use of azathioprine, NSAIDs and aspirin is covered in the sections on 'Rheumatoid arthritis' (earlier) and 'Antiphospholipid syndrome' (later).

■ Hydroxychloroquine should be continued since stopping may precipitate flare.

■ For control of hypertension, the drug of choice is methyldopa, with nifedipine or hydralazine as second-line agents (see chapter 1). Although long-term hydralazine and methyldopa use may rarely induce a SLE-like syndrome, they are not contraindicated in SLE.

Differentiation of active renal lupus from pre-eclampsia

■ This is notoriously difficult, and the two conditions may be superimposed.

■ Since hypertension, proteinuria, thrombocytopenia and even renal impairment are all features of pre-eclampsia, diagnosis of lupus flare requires other features, such as:
  – Rising anti-DNA antibody titre
  – Red blood cells or cellular casts in the urinary sediment
  – Fall in complement levels (elevation of complement split products, particularly Ba and Bb, often accompanies flares so high ratios of CH50:Ba may differentiate pre-eclamptics from those with active lupus)
  – Other symptoms of generalised flare, e.g. rashes or arthralgia.

■ Hyperuricaemia and abnormal liver function tests point more towards pre-eclampsia.

■ The only definitive investigation to reliably differentiate a renal lupus flare from pre-eclampsia is renal biopsy, but this is rarely undertaken in pregnancy. It is more likely to be appropriate prior to fetal viability, since confirmation of active lupus nephritis allows immunosuppressive treatment of the SLE without delivery.

■ If lupus flare and pre-eclampsia cannot be differentiated beyond 24–28 weeks' gestation, when the fetus is viable, delivery may be the most appropriate course if the mother or her fetus is at risk. Delivery will both cure pre-eclampsia and allow administration of drugs such as cyclophosphamide for a renal flare.

Neonatal lupus syndromes

■ These conditions are models of passively acquired autoimmunity. Autoantibodies directed against cytoplasmic ribonucleoproteins Ro and La cross the placenta, causing immune system damage to the fetus.

■ Several clinical syndromes have been described, of which cutaneous neonatal lupus is the most common, and congenital heart block (CHB) is the most serious. These syndromes rarely coexist.

■ More than 90% of mothers of affected offspring have anti-Ro antibodies, and 50–70% have anti-La antibodies. The prevalence of anti-Ro in the general population is <1%, although anti-Ro is present in about 30% of patients with SLE, commonly associated with photosensitivity, Sjögren's syndrome, subacute lupus erythematosus and ANA-negative SLE.

■ The risk of transient cutaneous lupus is only about 5% and the risk of CHB about 2% of the babies of Ro-positive mothers.

■ The risk of neonatal lupus is increased if a previous child has been affected, rising to 16% with one affected child and 50% if two children are affected; subsequent infants tend to be affected in the same way as their sibling.

■ Not all Ro-positive mothers of neonates with CHB have SLE; some have Sjögren's syndrome, some Raynaud's phenomenon or a photosensitive rash, and a large proportion are asymptomatic, although they may subsequently develop a connective tissue disease.

■ There is no correlation between the severity of maternal disease and the incidence of neonatal lupus, but mothers of babies with neonatal lupus do have a higher frequency of HLA-DR3, often with A1, B8.

Cutaneous form of neonatal lupus

■ This usually manifests in the first 2 weeks of life.

■ The infant develops typical geographical skin lesions similar to those of adult subacute cutaneous lupus, usually of the face and scalp, which appear after exposure to the sun.

■ The rash disappears spontaneously within 6 months, suggesting a direct antibody-mediated mechanism.

■ Residual hypopigmentation or telangiectasia may persist for up to 2 years, but scarring is unusual.

■ Sunlight and phototherapy should be avoided.

Congenital heart block (CHB)

- In contrast to cutaneous neonatal lupus, CHB appears *in utero*, is permanent, and may be fatal.

- The mechanism is not fully understood and no appropriate animal model exists. Reports of discordant twins suggest that fetal as well as maternal factors are involved.

- Although the fetal circulation is established by 12 weeks' gestation, CHB is not usually detected until 18–30 weeks' gestation. Once a fetal bradycardia is recognised, detailed scanning of the fetal heart, showing atrioventricular dissociation, confirms CHB.

- The pathogenesis is thought to involve inflammation and fibrosis of the conducting system. Other cardiac tissues may be affected, and a pancarditis with myocarditis and pericardial effusion may accompany the CHB. This is supported by the demonstration of binding of IgG anti-Ro antibodies to fetal hearts.

- There is no treatment that reverses CHB, although salbutamol given to the mother may be beneficial to the fetus if the bradycardia is causing fetal heart failure. This therapy may be limited by maternal side effects.

- If the fetal heart failure is thought to be due to myocarditis, dexamethasone and plasmapheresis may be successfully used, but these too have no effect on the conduction defect.

- The perinatal mortality rate is increased, with 19% of affected children dying in the early neonatal period. However, most infants who survive this period do well, although 50–60% require pacemakers in early infancy. All should be paced by their early teens to avoid the risk of sudden death.

Systemic lupus erythematosus – points to remember

- There is an increased rate of flare during pregnancy.
- Disease flares must be actively managed with corticosteroids.
- Adverse pregnancy outcome is related to the presence of renal involvement, hypertension, antiphospholipid antibodies and disease activity at the time of conception.
- These factors increase the risks of spontaneous miscarriage, fetal death, pre-eclampsia, preterm delivery and IUGR.
- Pregnancy care is best undertaken in combined clinics allowing close monitoring of disease activity, fetal growth and well-being.
- In Ro-positive mothers, the risk of transient neonatal cutaneous lupus is about 5% and the risk of CHB about 2%.

Antiphospholipid syndrome (APS)

Anticardiolipin antibodies (aCL) and lupus anticoagulant (LA) are overlapping subsets of antiphospholipid antibodies (aPL). The combination of either of these with one or more of the characteristic clinical features (Table 8.1) is known as the antiphospholipid syndrome (APS). Table 8.2 presents other features of APS.

Incidence

- ▪ It was first described in patients with SLE, but it is now recognised both that most patients with APS do not fulfil the diagnostic criteria for SLE and that those with primary APS do not usually progress to SLE.

Table 8.1 – Clinical criteria for the diagnosis of APS

Thrombosis	Venous Arterial Small vessel
Pregnancy morbidity	≥3 consecutive miscarriages (<10 weeks' gestation) ≥1 fetal death (>10 weeks' gestation with fetal heart documented) ≥1 premature birth (<34 weeks' gestation) due to pre-eclampsia or placental insufficiency

Table 8.2 – Other recognised features of APS

Thrombocytopenia	
Haemolytic anaemia	
Livedo reticularis	
Cerebral involvement	Epilepsy, cerebral infarction, chorea and migraine, transverse myelopathy/myelitis
Heart valve disease	Particularly mitral valve
Hypertension	
Pulmonary hypertension	
Leg ulcers	

■ The prevalence of aPL in the general obstetric population is low (<2%).

■ About 30% of women with SLE have aPL.

■ About 30% of those with aPL have thrombosis.

■ Up to 30% of women with severe early-onset pre-eclampsia may have aPL.

Clinical features

Although the clinical features of primary and SLE-associated APS are similar, and the antibody specificity is the same, the distinction is important, and patients with primary APS should not be labelled as having lupus.

Pathogenesis

■ The binding of aCL to cardiolipin requires the presence of a co-factor, β_2-glycoprotein (β_2GPI). This co-factor, an endogenous coagulation inhibitor, plays a key role in APS-associated thrombosis.

■ In APS-associated fetal loss, there is typically massive infarction and thrombosis of the placental and decidual vessels, probably secondary to spiral artery vasculopathy. Platelet deposition and prostanoid imbalance may be implicated in a similar way to pre-eclampsia.

■ Many of the adverse outcomes described are the end result of defective or abnormal placentation and these findings support placental failure, being the mechanism by which aPL is associated with late loss. But aCL-associated thrombosis within the placenta cannot explain all the recognised pregnancy complications in APS.

■ aPL bind to human trophoblasts *in vitro*. Trophoblast cell membranes behave as targets for both β_2GPI-dependent and β_2GPI-independent aPL.

■ aPL reduce hCG release and inhibit trophoblast invasiveness.

Diagnosis

■ Firm diagnosis of APS requires two or more positive readings for LA and/or aCL at least 8 weeks apart, plus at least one of the clinical criteria listed in Table 8.1.

■ Lupus anticoagulant is a misnomer coined because it prolongs coagulation times *in vitro*. It is detected by the prolongation of the activated partial thromboplastin time (aPTT) or the dilute Russell's viper venom time (dRVVT). This prolongation fails to correct with the addition of platelet poor plasma, but corrects with excess phospholipid.

■ Anticardiolipin antibodies are measured using commercially available enzyme-linked immunosorbent assay (ELISA) kits. Medium or high titres of IgG or IgM are required.

Pregnancy

Effect of pregnancy on APS

▪ The risk of thrombosis is exacerbated by the hypercoagulable pregnant state.

▪ Pre-existing thrombocytopenia may worsen.

Effect of APS on pregnancy

▪ The risks of miscarriage, second and third trimester fetal death, pre-eclampsia, IUGR, and placental abruption are increased.

▪ Establishing causality for first trimester losses is difficult, since the risk of miscarriage is high (10–15%) in the normal population. aPL are more common in women suffering three or more first-trimester miscarriages, than in those with one or two miscarriages.

▪ Fetal death in APS is typically preceded by IUGR and oligohydramnios.

▪ The risk of fetal loss is directly related to antibody titre, particularly the IgG aCL, although many women with a history of recurrent loss have only IgM antibodies.

▪ Quantifying the risk is difficult and the presence of aPL does not preclude successful pregnancy.

▪ Previous obstetric history is the best predictor of pregnancy outcome in women with APS.

▪ Reported outcomes vary depending on whether the study population is made up of those with predominantly recurrent miscarriage (in whom complications are less likely) or those with SLE, thrombosis or previous late intrauterine death (in whom the risk of premature delivery before 37 weeks' gestation exceeds 40% and the risk of IUGR exceeds 30%).

▪ Pre-eclampsia is common and often severe, and of early onset in the latter group.

Management

Pre-pregnancy

▪ Women with a history of thrombosis, recurrent miscarriage, intrauterine fetal death, or severe early-onset pre-eclampsia should be screened for the presence of LA or aCL.

▪ A detailed history of the circumstances of the fetal loss is essential to exclude other causes of late miscarriage, such as cervical incompetence or idiopathic premature labour. The presence of aPL does not constitute a diagnosis of APS unless the clinical features are suggestive.

Antenatal

- Care of pregnant women with APS should be multidisciplinary and in centres with expertise in the management of this condition.

- Aspirin inhibits thromboxane and may reduce the risk of vascular thrombosis. There are many non-randomised studies suggesting that low-dose aspirin is effective and it can prevent pregnancy loss in experimental APS mice.

- Randomised, controlled trials of aspirin as a single agent in APS pregnancy do not support any benefit over placebo, however such studies have been undertaken in low-risk women. Most centres now advocate treatment with low-dose aspirin for all women with APS, prior to conception, in the belief that the placental damage occurs early in gestation, and that aspirin may prevent failure of placentation.

- Women with APS and previous thromboembolism are at extremely high risk of further thromboembolism in pregnancy and the puerperium and should receive antenatal thromboprophylaxis with s.c. heparin. Most centres now use low-molecular-weight heparin (LMWH) (see chapter 3). Many of these women are on life-long anticoagulation therapy with warfarin. The change from warfarin to heparin should be achieved prior to 6 weeks' gestation to avoid warfarin embryopathy.

- A few women with cerebral arterial thrombosis due to APS on long-term warfarin may experience transient ischaemic symptoms when LMWH is substituted for warfarin. If these do not improve on higher doses of LMWH, the reintroduction of warfarin is justified to prevent maternal stroke.

- Opinion is divided about the best therapy for those with recurrent pregnancy loss, but without a history of thromboembolism.

- Treatment with high-dose steroids (in the absence of active lupus) to suppress LA and aCL, in combination with aspirin, is no longer recommended because of the maternal side effects from such prolonged high doses of steroids. This strategy has been abandoned in favour of anticoagulant treatment with aspirin and/or s.c. heparin or LMWH. Such regimens give equivalent fetal outcome with fewer maternal side effects than combinations of aspirin and steroids.

- Any additional benefit of heparin must be balanced against the risk of heparin-induced osteoporosis (likely to be low with LMWHs), and the cost and inconvenience of daily injections.

- In women with recurrent miscarriage, but without a history of thrombosis, aspirin and LMWH improves the live birth rate compared to aspirin alone. However this improvement is due solely to a decrease in the risk of miscarriage before 13 weeks' gestation. More recent data do not confirm a beneficial effect for LMWH over and above aspirin.

- Antithrombotic strategies vary in different centres around the world. A suggested protocol is given in Table 8.3.

- LMWH is given in prophylactic doses (enoxaparin [Clexane®] 40 mg o.d; dalteparin [Fragmin®] 5000 units o.d.), except for women with previous thrombosis where higher doses (e.g. dalteparin [Fragmin®] 5000 units b.d.), may be indicated.

Table 8.3 – Therapeutic management of APS pregnancies

Clinical history	Anticoagulant therapy
No thrombosis, no miscarriage, no adverse pregnancy outcome	Aspirin 75 mg o.d. from pre-conception
Previous thrombosis	*On maintenance warfarin:* transfer to aspirin and LMWH as soon as pregnancy confirmed *Not on warfarin:* aspirin 75 mg o.d. from pre-conception and commence LMWH once pregnancy confirmed
Recurrent miscarriage <10 weeks only	*No prior anticoagulant therapy:* Aspirin 75 mg o.d. from pre-conception *Prior miscarriage with aspirin alone:* Aspirin 75 mg o.d. from pre-conception and LMWH once pregnancy confirmed. Consider discontinuation of LWWH at 20 weeks' gestation if uterine artery waveform is normal
Late fetal loss, neonatal death or adverse outcome due to pre-eclampsia, IUGR or abruption	Aspirin 75 mg o.d. from pre-conception and LMWH once pregnancy confirmed

■ Immunosuppression with azathioprine, i.v. immunoglobulin (IVIg) and plasmapheresis have all been tried. The numbers treated do not allow firm conclusions regarding efficacy, although there is some evidence of this sort available for IVIg. IVIg is extremely expensive, precluding its use outside a research setting in most centres.

■ Close fetal monitoring is essential. Uterine artery Doppler waveform analysis at 20–24 weeks' gestation helps predict the higher risk pregnancies. Monthly growth scans and umbilical artery Doppler blood flow are performed from 28 weeks (or 24 weeks if the uterine artery Doppler waveform at 24 weeks shows pre-diastolic 'notching').

■ High-risk women require closer surveillance with regular blood pressure checks and urinalysis to detect early-onset pre-eclampsia.

■ Such intensive monitoring allows for timely delivery, which may improve fetal outcome.

Postpartum

■ Women on long-term warfarin treatment may recommence this postpartum (starting days 2–3) and LMWH is discontinued when the international normalised ratio (INR) is >2.0.

- Women with previous thrombosis should receive postpartum heparin or warfarin for 6 weeks.
- Women without previous thrombosis should receive postpartum heparin for 5 days.

Antiphospholipid syndrome – points to remember

- Not all women with APS have SLE.
- The important clinical features are recurrent miscarriage, intrauterine fetal death, and thrombosis.
- Even in the absence of fetal loss, there is an increased risk of severe, early onset pre-eclampsia, IUGR, and placental abruption.
- Previous poor obstetric history is the most important predictor of fetal loss.
- Management should be multidisciplinary in centres with expertise in APS and with facilities for regular and close fetal surveillance.
- Treatment is with low-dose aspirin with or without LMWH.

Scleroderma

Incidence

This is rare (2.3–12 cases per million per year) but more common in women (female to male ratio 3:1).

Clinical features

- Scleroderma may be divided into:
  - Localised cutaneous form (morphoea) with areas of waxy, thickened skin, usually on the forearms and hands
  - Systemic sclerosis associated with Raynaud's phenomenon and organ involvement
  - CREST syndrome (calcinosis, Raynaud's phenomenon, oesophageal involvement, sclerodactyly, telangiectasia).
- The skin in systemic sclerosis is typically bound down to produce sclerodactyly, beaking of the nose, a fixed facial expression and limitation of mouth opening. Skin ulceration and partial digit amputation are common.
- Systemic involvement usually takes the form of progressive fibrosis and includes the oesophagus most commonly (80%), lungs (45%), heart (40%) and kidneys (35%).

Pathogenesis and immunology

- The aetiology is unknown.
- There may be associated antinuclear, anticentromere (CREST), antinucleolar or SCL-70 antibodies.

Pregnancy

Effect of pregnancy on scleroderma

- The prognosis for localised cutaneous scleroderma without organ involvement is good.
- Those with early diffuse systemic sclerosis (<4 years) and/or renal involvement are at risk of rapid overall deterioration and renal crisis during pregnancy.
- Raynaud's disease tends to improve as a result of vasodilation and increased blood flow.
- Reflux oesophagitis may deteriorate due to lowered oesophageal tone.
- Those with severe pulmonary fibrosis and pulmonary hypertension are at high risk of postpartum deterioration.

Effect of scleroderma on pregnancy

- Overall success rates are 70–80%.
- There is an increased risk of premature delivery. Late diffuse disease is associated with an increased risk of miscarriage.
- Pre-eclampsia, IUGR and perinatal mortality are risks for women with hypertension and renal disease.
- Venepuncture, venous access and blood pressure measurement may be difficult because of skin or blood vessel involvement.
- General anaesthesia may be complicated by difficult endotracheal intubation, and regional anaesthesia may also be difficult.

Management

- No treatment has been shown to influence the progress of scleroderma and management is therefore symptomatic.
- Women should be advised to delay pregnancy until the disease has stabilised.
- Pre-pregnancy assessment with formal lung function tests and echocardiography is important.
- Women with multiple or severe organ involvement (pulmonary hypertension, severe pulmonary fibrosis, renal involvement) should be advised against pregnancy.

- Raynaud's phenomenon may be helped by heated gloves or nifedipine, which may be used safely in pregnancy.
- Regular multidisciplinary assessment for disease activity, fetal well-being and blood pressure checks are essential.
- Although generally contraindicated in pregnancy, the benefits of angiotensin-inhibiting enzyme (ACE) inhibitors in scleroderma renal crisis outweigh the risks to the fetus, and their use is justified in this situation.
- Early assessment by an anaesthetist is advisable if problems with regional or general anaesthesia are anticipated.
- Steroid treatment should be avoided as this may precipitate a renal crisis.
- β_2-agonists should be avoided for preterm labour because of their vasoconstrictive action.

Ehlers–Danlos syndrome (EDS)

- This group of disorders consists of inherited (predominantly autosomal dominant) defects of collagen metabolism, characterised by fragile skin and blood vessels, easy bruising, skin hyperelasticity and joint hypermobility.
- Types I (classic or gravis) and IV (ecchymotic or arterial) carry the highest risks in pregnancy, and maternal mortality with type IV may be as high as 20–25%.
- Types II (mitis) and X (fibronectin abnormality) have more favourable outcomes.

Pregnancy

Effect of EDS on pregnancy

Problems in pregnancy arise mostly at delivery and include:
- Spontaneous vaginal, perineal and other visceral tears
- Skin fragility and poor healing
- Great vessel rupture
- Uterine rupture
- Postpartum haemorrhage (common)
- Increased risk of premature rupture of membranes, malpresentation
- Increased risk of IUGR.

Management

- Preconceptual categorisation of disorder and genetic counselling is essential.
- Avoidance or termination of pregnancy is advisable for those with type IV.
- Caesarean section may not result in fewer complications.

Pregnancy-associated osteoporosis

Incidence

- Normal pregnancy is associated with a significant fall in bone density, and rarely idiopathic transient osteoporosis of pregnancy may develop.
- Osteoporosis is defined as bone density <2.5 standard deviations below the mean for young adults.

Clinical features

- Presentation is with hip joint or most frequently back pain usually during the third trimester or puerperium of the first full-term pregnancy.
- Bone mineral density usually recovers within a year after delivery, although may be delayed until the cessation of lactation and recurrence in subsequent pregnancies is mild or absent.
- There is no correlation between bone mass and parity, suggesting full recovery between pregnancies.

Pathogenesis

- Reduction in bone density affects trabecular rather than cortical bone.
- Osteoporosis results from either excessive osteoclastic activity with accelerated bone resorption and remodelling, or decreased osteoblastic activity.
- Osteoporosis may stem from a failure in the changes of calcitropic hormones (vitamin D, calcitonin and parathyroid hormone [PTH]) to cope with the increased demand for calcium in pregnancy.
- The condition may represent pre-existing osteopenia (bone density between 1 and 2.5 standard deviation [SD] below mean) and a low peak bone mass that is unmasked and becomes symptomatic during pregnancy. The latter may be a result of additional mechanical stresses or simply an exaggeration of the physiological changes that occur in bone during pregnancy and lactation.
- Continued lactation may exacerbate the problem, causing a further reduction on bone density, but it is unlikely to be the primary aetiological influence.
- Studies suggest an uncoupling of bone formation and bone resorption in the latter half of pregnancy. Although both increase in pregnancy, the rate of bone resorption exceeds the rate of bone formation.
- An aetiological role for PTH-related peptide is also suggested.

Diagnosis

Radiological (if postpartum) or ultrasound or dual X-ray absorptiometry (DXA) investigations show signs of demineralisation of the femoral head or lumbar spine (80% trabecular bone) with non-traumatic compression vertebral fractures in severe cases.

Management

This usually requires avoidance of weightbearing to prevent pain and fractures.

Further reading

Janssen, N.M. and Genta, M.S. (2000) The effects of immunosuppressive and anti-inflammatory medications on fertility, pregnancy, and lactation. *Arch. Intern. Med.*, **160,** 610–619.

Khamashta, M.A., Cuadrado, M.J., Mujic, F., Taub, N.A., Hunt, B.J. and Hughes, G.R. (1995) The management of thrombosis in the antiphospholipid-antibody syndrome. *N. Engl. J. Med.*, **332,** 993–997.

Khamashta, M.A., Ruiz-Irastoza, G. and Hughes, G.R.V. (1997) Systemic lupus erythematosus flares during pregnancy. *Rheum. Dis. Clin. North Am.*, **23,** 15–30.

Langford, K. and Nelson-Piercy, C. (1999). Antiphospholipid syndrome in pregnancy. *Contemp. Rev. Obstet. Gynaecol.*, **6,** 93–98.

Lima, F., Khamashta, M.A., Buchanan, N.M.M., Kerstake, S., Hunt, B.J. and Hughes, G.R.V. (1996). A study of sixty pregnancies in patients with the antiphospholipid syndrome. *Clin. Exp. Rheumatol.*, **14,** 131–136.

Ostenson, M. and Ramsey-Goldman, R. (1998). Treatment of inflammatory rheumatic disorders in pregnancy. *Drug Safety* **19,** 389–410.

Oviasu, E., Hicks, J. and Cameron, J.S. (1991) The outcome of pregnancy in women with lupus nephritis. *Lupus*, **1,** 19–25.

Nelson, J.L. and Ostensen, M. (1997). Pregnancy and rheumatoid arthritis. *Rheum. Dis. Clin. North Am.*, **23,** 195–212.

Smith, R., Athanasou, N.A., Ostlere, S.J. and Vipond, S.E. (1995) Pregnancy-associated osteoporosis. *QJM*, **88,** 865–878.

Steen, V.D. (1999) Pregnancy in women with systemic sclerosis. *Obstet. Gynecol.*, **94,** 15–20.

Waltuck, J. and Buyon, J.P. (1994) Autoantibody-associated congenital heart block: outcome in mothers and children. *Ann. Intern. Med.*, **120,** 544–551.

CHAPTER 9

Neurological problems

Epilepsy	Stroke
Migraine and headache	Ischaemic stroke
Multiple sclerosis	Intracerebral haemorrhage
Myasthenia gravis	Haemorrhagic stroke
Myotonic dystrophy	Subarachnoid haemorrhage
Benign intracranial hypertension	Bell's palsy
Cerebral vein thrombosis	

Epilepsy

Incidence

Epilepsy affects about 0.5% of women of child-bearing age and is the commonest chronic neurological disorder to complicate pregnancy.

Clinical features

Epilepsy is classified according to the clinical type of seizures and whether they are partial or generalised. The most common are as follows:

- Tonic–clonic seizure (grand mal)
- Absence seizure (petit mal)
- Temporal lobe seizures (complex partial seizure)
- Myoclonic seizure.

Absence seizures (petit mal) typically have a short duration, a rapid onset without warning and a rapid recovery. They are associated with 3 Hz spike-and-wave discharge on the electroencephalogram (EEG).

Pathogenesis

Most cases of epilepsy are idiopathic and no underlying cause is found. About 30% of these patients have a family history of epilepsy.

Secondary epilepsy may be encountered in pregnancy in patients who have the following:

- Previous surgery to the cerebral hemispheres
- Intracranial mass lesions (meningiomas and arteriovenous malformations enlarge during pregnancy. This should always be considered if the first seizure occurs in pregnancy)
- Antiphospholipid syndrome (see chapter 8, p. 146).

Other causes of seizures in pregnancy (see also Section B, Table 8) include the following:

- Eclampsia (see chapter 1, p. 8)
- Cerebral vein thrombosis (CVT) (see chapter 3, p. 57)
- Thrombotic thrombocytopenic purpura (TTP) (see chapter 14, p. 266)
- Cerebral infarction (risk is increased in pregnancy and 4% have seizures, see p. 174)
- Subarachnoid haemorrhage (see p. 176)
- Drug and alcohol withdrawal
- Hypoglycaemia (diabetes, hypoadrenalism, hypopituitarism, liver failure)
- Hypocalcaemia (magnesium sulphate therapy, hypoparathyroidism)
- Hyponatraemia (hyperemesis, hypoadrenalism)
- Postdural puncture. Seizures are rare and preceded by typical postdural puncture headache and other neurological symptoms. Seizures occur typically 4–7 days after dural puncture
- Gestational epilepsy (seizures are confined to pregnancy)
- Pseudoepilepsy (these patients usually have true epilepsy as well). Useful distinguishing features to differentiate these 'pseudo fits' are:
  – Prolonged/repeated seizures without cyanosis
  – Resistance to passive eye-opening
  – Down-going plantar reflexes
  – Persistence of a positive conjunctival reflex.

Diagnosis

Most women with epilepsy in pregnancy have already been diagnosed, but when a first seizure occurs in pregnancy, the following investigations are appropriate:

- Blood pressure, urinalysis, uric acid, platelet count, clotting screen, blood film
- Blood glucose, serum calcium, serum sodium, liver function tests
- Computerised tomography (CT) or magnetic resonance imaging (MRI) of the brain. Although this is not necessarily recommended for the first seizure in the non-pregnant woman, there is no doubt of its value in pregnancy, bearing in mind the above differential diagnoses.
- EEG.

Pregnancy

Effect of pregnancy on epilepsy

- About 25–30% of women experience an increased frequency of seizures in pregnancy.
- In most (54%), the frequency of seizures is not altered by pregnancy.
- A woman who has been seizure-free for many years is unlikely to have seizures in pregnancy unless she discontinues her medication.
- Those with poorly controlled epilepsy, especially those whose seizure frequency exceeds once a month, are more likely to deteriorate in pregnancy.
- There is no relation to the seizure type or course of epilepsy during previous pregnancies.
- Women with multiple seizure types are also more likely to experience an increase in seizure frequency in pregnancy.
- The risk of seizures is highest peripartum (see later).
- Epilepsy is the second commonest indirect cause of maternal death in the UK. There were 19 maternal deaths due to epilepsy from 1994–1996. Most of these deaths occurred antenatally in the third trimester. In 10 women the cause of death was aspiration, but epileptic seizures may be fatal in themselves. In only five women was the epilepsy poorly controlled and two died having had no seizure for 2 years prior to pregnancy. It may be that pregnancy increases the risk of sudden unexplained death in epilepsy (SUDEP) estimated at 1 in 500 woman-years outside pregnancy.

Possible reasons for deterioration in seizure control during pregnancy include:

- Pregnancy itself
- Poor compliance with anticonvulsant medication (due to fears regarding teratogenesis)
- Decreased drug levels related to nausea and vomiting in early pregnancy
- Decreased drug levels related to increased volume of distribution and increased drug clearance through the liver and kidney. Changes in protein binding will tend to increase the free level of drugs, but this is usually outweighed by the first two factors
- Lack of sleep towards term and during labour
- Lack of absorption of anticonvulsant drugs from the gastrointestinal tract during labour
- Hyperventilation during labour.

Effect of epilepsy on pregnancy

- The fetus is relatively resistant to short episodes of hypoxia and there is no evidence of adverse effects of single seizures on the fetus. Some have documented fetal bradycardia during and after maternal tonic–clonic convulsions, but cerebral damage in the long term is not a feature.

- There is no increased risk of miscarriage or obstetric complications in epileptics unless a seizure results in abdominal trauma.
- Status epilepticus is dangerous for both mother and fetus and should be treated vigorously. Fortunately this complicates <1% of pregnancies in epileptics.
- The main concern stems from the increased risk of congenital abnormalities (see later). Even children of epileptics (fathers and mothers) who are not taking any anticonvulsants have a slightly increased risk (4%) compared to the general population (3%).
- The risk of the child developing epilepsy is also increased (5%) if either parent has epilepsy.
- If there is a previously affected sibling, the risk is 10%.
- If both parents have epilepsy, the risk is 15–20%.
- The risk of a patient with idiopathic generalised epilepsy having an affected child is about 9–12%. For those with partial seizures, the risk is lower (3%).

Teratogenic risks of anticonvulsants

- Phenytoin, primidone, phenobarbitone, carbamazepine and sodium valproate all cross the placenta and are teratogenic.
- The major malformations caused by anticonvulsants are:
  - Neural tube defects (particularly valproate [1–2%] and carbamazepine [0.5–1%])
  - Orofacial clefts (particularly phenytoin)
  - Congenital heart defects (particularly phenytoin and valproate).
- Minor malformations (fetal anticonvulsant syndrome) associated with anticonvulsant use in pregnancy include:
  - Dysmorphic features (V-shaped eyebrows, low-set ears, broad nasal bridge, irregular teeth)
  - Hypertelorism
  - Hypoplastic nails and distal digits.
- There is little difference in the level of risk between individual drugs.
- The risk for any one drug is about 6–7% (i.e. two- to three-fold the background level of risk).
- The risk increases with the number of drugs, so for those taking two or more anticonvulsants, the risk is 15%; for those taking the combination of valproate, carbamazepine and phenytoin, the risk is as high as 50%.
- For valproate there is evidence of a dose-dependent teratogenic effect. Offspring of mothers using >1 g/day are at a six-fold increased risk of congenital malformations, particularly neural tube defects, compared to those exposed to 600 mg/day or less.

■ One mechanism for teratogenesis is thought to be folate deficiency. Phenytoin and phenobarbitone particularly, but also carbamazepine and valproate, interfere with folate metabolism.

■ The risk of neural tube and also cardiovascular and urogenital defects, and oral clefts is likely to be decreased by the use of pre-conceptual and first-trimester folic acid.

■ The newer anticonvulsant drugs lamotrigine, gabapentin and tiagabine are not teratogenic in animals. Few data of their use in human pregnancy exist, but the risk of malformations with lamotrigine seems no higher than the other principal anti-epileptic drugs.

■ Animal studies have shown a teratogenic risk for vigabatrin and topiramate.

■ The benzodiazepines (e.g. clonazepam) are not teratogenic.

Management

Antenatal management in established epilepsy

■ All women receiving anticonvulsant drugs should be advised to take folic acid 5 mg daily for at least 12 weeks prior to conception. This should be continued throughout pregnancy as there is also a small risk of folate-deficiency anaemia.

■ There is no need to change the anticonvulsant in pregnancy if the woman is well controlled with phenytoin, carbamazepine, valproate, or lamotrigine. Phenobarbitone may be weaned or changed (under close supervision) to a different drug since there is a risk of neonatal withdrawal convulsions.

■ Sodium valproate therapy should be changed to a three or four times daily regimen or a modified-release preparation to lower peak concentrations and reduce the risk of neural tube defects. Slow-release preparations of valproate (Epilim chrono®) and carbamazepine (Tegretol retard®) also seem to give better control during pregnancy.

■ Relatives, friends and/or partners should be advised on how to place the woman in the recovery position to prevent aspiration in the event of a seizure.

■ Women should be advised to bathe in shallow water or to shower.

■ Pre-natal screening for congenital abnormalities with nuchal translucency scanning and detailed ultrasound at 18–20 weeks should be offered. A repeat scan (preferably by a fetal cardiologist) at 22 weeks is advisable if cardiac defects are suspected.

■ The altered pharmocokinetics in pregnancy mean that drug levels are likely to change, and for most drugs, concentration of the free drug falls.

■ A baseline serum or salivary drug level is useful to establish compliance and inform future changes in drug doses.

■ If a woman is seizure-free, there is no need to measure drug levels serially or adjust the dose unless she has a seizure.

- In women who have regular seizures and who are dependent on critical drug levels, it is worth monitoring drug levels since they are likely to fall, and increasing doses of anticonvulsants should be guided by serum concentrations of the free drug.
- In general it is preferable to be guided by the patient and her seizure frequency rather than by drug levels.
- If corticosteroids are administered to induce fetal lung maturity, it should be remembered that higher doses are required in women receiving hepatic enzyme-inducing drugs (carbamazepine, phenytoin, phenobarbitone).
- Vitamin K (10–20 mg orally) should be prescribed in the last 4 weeks of pregnancy for epileptic women taking hepatic enzyme-inducing drugs. This is because in babies of women receiving these drugs, vitamin K-dependent clotting factors may be reduced and the risk of haemorrhagic disease of the newborn is increased.

Intrapartum management

- The risk of seizures increases around the time of delivery.
- 1–2% of women with epilepsy will have a seizure during labour and 1–2% will have one in the first 24 hours postpartum.
- The woman should continue her regular anti-epileptic drugs in labour.
- If there is particular concern regarding a high risk of intrapartum seizures, then carbamazepine can be administered rectally, or phenytoin can be given intravenously.
- To limit the risk of precipitating a seizure due to pain and anxiety, early epidural analgesia should be considered.
- I.v. lorazepam is an appropriate acute treatment for serial seizures in labour.
- Most women with epilepsy have normal vaginal deliveries and caesarean section is only required if there are recurrent generalised seizures in late pregnancy or labour.

Postnatal management

- The neonate should also receive 1 mg vitamin K intramuscularly.
- All women with epilepsy should be encouraged to breast-feed. Most anticonvulsants are secreted into breast milk, but the dose received by the baby is only a fraction of the therapeutic level for neonates, and in any case is less than that received *in utero*.
- Babies whose mothers received phenobarbitone in pregnancy may experience withdrawal symptoms if they are not breast-fed, and although this is rare with the newer anticonvulsants, it provides a logical reason to encourage breast-feeding in all epileptic mothers.

- Approximate transfers from plasma to breast milk are:
  - phenytoin   18–20%
  - carbamazepine   40%
  - sodium valproate   1–10%
  - lamotrigine   40–45%

The largest amounts of drug likely to be received by an infant, expressed as a percentage of the recommended therapeutic dose are:
  - phenytoin   5%
  - carbamazepine   5%
  - sodium valproate   3%
  - phenobarbitone   50%

Phenobarbitone, primidone and lamotrigine can accumulate in a breast-fed baby due to slow elimination.

- If the mother's dose of anticonvulsant was increased during pregnancy, it may be gradually decreased again over a few weeks in the puerperium. Blood levels of phenytoin increase rapidly following delivery, but carbamazepine and valproate take longer to return to pre-conception levels.

- If a baby of a mother taking anticonvulsants is unusually sleepy or has to be woken for feeds, the mother should be encouraged to feed before rather than after taking her anticonvulsants. This should avoid peak serum and therefore breast-milk levels.

- The mother should be advised of strategies to minimise the risk to her baby should she have a seizure. This includes changing nappies with the baby on the floor and bathing the baby in very shallow water or with supervision.

Management of newly diagnosed idiopathic epilepsy in pregnancy

- The annual incidence of new cases of epilepsy in women of child-bearing age is 20–30 per 100 000.

- Having excluded all the secondary causes of seizures listed earlier, it is not obligatory to treat one isolated seizure.

- If treatment is required, carbamazepine, valproate and lamotrigine are reasonable choices. However, the type of epilepsy guides anticonvulsant therapy, and generalised seizures with myoclonus and photosensitivity respond particularly well to sodium valproate.

Pre-pregnancy counselling

- Ideally, this should form part of the routine management of epilepsy in pregnancy.

- It should be assumed that all women of child-bearing age may become pregnant and therefore any opportunity to counsel such women should be taken.

■ Control of epilepsy should be maximised prior to pregnancy with the lowest dose of the most effective treatment that gives best seizure control. Polytherapy should be avoided if possible.

■ Review of anticonvulsant medication should take into account the risk of teratogenesis. If there are any issues concerning fertility, it is important to remember the association between sodium valproate and polycystic ovarian syndrome.

■ Any changes to minimise the risk of neural tube defects (e.g. a decrease in the dose of sodium valproate) should be made pre-conception since the neural tube closes at gestational day 26.

■ Women who have been seizure-free for more than 2 years may wish to discontinue anticonvulsants at least pre-conceptually and for the first trimester. This should be a fully informed decision after counselling concerning particularly the risk of losing a driving licence in the event of a seizure. The risk of a seizure within the first year after discontinuation of anti-epileptic drugs in a woman who has been seizure-free for 2 or more years is 20%.

■ The current recommendations are to stop driving from the commencement of the period of drug withdrawal and for a period of 6 months after cessation of treatment, even if there is no recurrence of seizures.

■ All women on anticonvulsant drugs should be advised to take preconceptual folic acid (5 mg/day).

Contraception

■ Women taking hepatic enzyme-inducing drugs (phenytoin, primidone, carbamazepine, phenobarbitone) require higher doses of oestrogen to achieve adequate contraception. They should be given a combined oral contraceptive pill containing 50 μg ethinyloestradiol. If breakthrough bleeding occurs, the dose should be increased to 75 or 100 μg. The combined oral contraceptive pill may still not be effective and an alternative method of contraception may be appropriate.

■ The efficacy of the progesterone-only pill is also affected by enzyme-inducing anti-epileptic medication. Women should be advised not to rely solely on this method.

■ Medroxyprogesterone injections (Depot-Provera®) are effective and larger doses are not needed since elimination is dependent on hepatic first-pass rather than enzyme activity.

■ The 'morning after pill' can be used if required but a slightly higher dose may be needed.

■ The levonorgestrel implant has a very high failure rate in these women.

■ Valproate, clonazepam, vigabatrin, lamotrigine and gabapentin do not induce hepatic enzymes and all methods of contraception are suitable.

Epilepsy – points to remember

■ All women receiving anti-epileptic drugs should receive pre-pregnancy counselling and be advised to take folic acid 5 mg daily pre-conceptually.

■ Most anticonvulsant drugs are teratogenic. The risk is lower with mono- rather than polytherapy.

■ Prenatal screening for congenital abnormalities should be offered.

■ In most women, the frequency of seizures is not altered by pregnancy provided there is compliance with anti-epileptic drug regimens.

■ Free drug levels tend to fall in pregnancy and increased doses of anti-epileptic drugs may be required.

■ Vitamin K (10–20 mg orally daily) should be prescribed for all epileptic women in the last 4 weeks of pregnancy.

■ Breast-feeding should be encouraged.

■ Hepatic enzyme-inducing drugs reduce the efficacy of most hormonal methods of contraception, particularly the combined oral contraceptive pill.

Migraine and headache

Incidence

■ This is a common problem in pregnancy.

■ Differentiation between tension headache and migraine can be very difficult and not all migraine is 'classical'.

■ Migraine can occur and worsen in pregnancy in known migraine sufferers. It may also occur as a pregnancy-related phenomenon in women without any prior history of migrainous headaches.

■ Migraine and headache account for almost one-third of neurological problems encountered in pregnancy.

Clinical features

■ Features of a headache that make migraine a likely diagnosis are the following:
   – Throbbing, unilateral headache
   – Prodromal symptoms that are usually visual, including scotoma, teichopsia and fortification spectra
   – Nausea and vomiting
   – Photophobia.

- During the prodromal phase of classical migraine, transient hemianopia, aphasia and sensory symptoms may occur. In hemiplegic migraine, the hemiparesis may last several hours and differentiation from a transient ischaemic attack is difficult.
- Hemiplegic migraine may rarely lead to cerebral infarction.
- Migraine associated with such focal signs may occur in up to 0.1% of pregnancies.
- Most cases occur in the third trimester and 40% occur in women with no previous history of migraine.

Pathogenesis

- Tension headaches are thought to be due to muscle contraction and are often related to periods of stress.
- Migraine is thought to be due to vasodilation of cerebral blood vessels, possibly related to platelet aggregation and serotonin (5-hydroxytryptamine [5-HT]) release with stimulation of nociceptors.
- Migraine may be precipitated by:
  - Certain dietary factors (e.g. chocolate, cheese)
  - Premenstruation
  - Oral contraceptive pill
  - Stress.

Diagnosis

- Diagnosis is made by taking a careful history and performing a neurological examination (in order to exclude focal signs, neck stiffness, and papilloedema).
- Any focal signs lasting longer than 24 hours warrant further investigation with cerebral imaging. There is no test to confirm the diagnosis of migraine.
- The differential diagnosis (see also Section B, Table 7) of headache in pregnancy and the puerperium includes:
  - Pre-eclampsia
  - Postdural puncture headache
  - Sub-arachnoid haemorrhage
  - Meningitis
  - Cerebral vein thrombosis
  - Benign intracranial hypertension
  - Intracranial mass lesions.

Pregnancy

Effect of pregnancy on migraine

- 50–90% of women with pre-existing classical migraine improve during pregnancy.

- Improvement is most marked in the second and third trimesters.
- Improvement is more common in those with premenstrual migraine.
- Migraine may present for the first time during pregnancy.

Management

- For the acute attack, paracetamol-based analgesics with or without anti-emetics (e.g. metoclopramide, buclizine, cyclizine) are used.
- Codeine phosphate is also safe for use in pregnancy.
- Ergotamine is contraindicated.
- Sumatriptan (Imigran®), a 5-HT_1 agonist is commonly used in non-pregnant women for control of acute attacks. There are limited data of its use in pregnancy and it is usually avoided, although there is no evidence of it causing major defects.
- Prophylaxis should be considered if attacks are longlasting or frequent.
- Low-dose aspirin (75 mg daily) is safe and effective for prophylaxis of migraine complicating pregnancy, and should be considered as a first-line agent.
- β-blockers (propranolol 10–40 mg t.d.s.) are reserved for resistant cases without contraindications. These work in >80% of patients. The use of β-blockers throughout pregnancy has been associated with growth restriction (see chapter 1, p. 14).
- If both aspirin and β-blockers are ineffective in preventing headache and migraine in pregnancy, then tricyclic antidepressants such as amitriptyline (25–50 mg at night) or calcium antagonists may prove useful and are safe for use in pregnancy.
- There are few data regarding pizotifen (Sanomigran®), a serotonin antagonist used for prevention of migraine outside pregnancy, but its use is justified after the first trimester if first- and second-line prophylactic agents are not effective.

Contraception

Women with classical migraine should not take oestrogen-containing oral contraceptives.

Migraine – points to remember

- Migraine can occur as a pregnancy-related phenomenon in women without prior history of migraine.
- Those with pre-existing migraine often improve in pregnancy.
- Hemiplegic migraine may mimic transient ischaemic attacks (TIAs).
- Ergotamine should be avoided in pregnancy.
- Low-dose aspirin, β-blockers, tricyclic antidepressants, and pizotifen may be used for prophylaxis.

Multiple sclerosis (MS)

Incidence

This disease is relatively common (0.06–0.1% in the UK) with the typical age of onset during the child-bearing years.

Clinical features

- MS typically runs a relapsing and remitting clinical course.
- Common presentations include optic neuritis, diplopia, sensory symptoms or weakness of the limbs.
- The course of MS is extremely variable; some are perfectly normal between relapses, others have severe disabilities.

Pathogenesis

- The cause is not known and prevalence is higher with increasing latitude, so the condition is uncommon in equatorial regions.
- There are multiple areas of demyelination within the brain and spinal cord.

Diagnosis

- There is no single diagnostic test. Most patients encountered in pregnancy are aware of their diagnosis.
- Cerebrospinal fluid examination, visually evoked responses, and MRI are all used to help confirm the diagnosis.

Pregnancy

Effect of pregnancy on MS

- MS is less likely to present for the first time and less likely to relapse during pregnancy.
- The decrease in relapse rate during pregnancy is most marked in the third trimester, and accompanied by cessation of disease activity on MRI. This is possibly related to the decrease in cell-mediated immunity and the increase in humoral immunity characteristic of pregnancy.
- Those with neuropathic bladders may experience increased problems with urinary tract infection during pregnancy.
- The rate of relapse increases markedly in the first 3 months postpartum, but declines to pre-pregnant levels by 10 months after delivery.
- Exacerbation during the 3–6 months following delivery occurs in up to 40% of patients.
- Neither breast-feeding nor epidural analgesia have an adverse effect on the rate of relapse.
- The overall rate of progression of disability is not altered by pregnancy.
- There is no long-term effect of pregnancy or breast-feeding on the course of MS.

Effect of MS on pregnancy

There is little effect of MS on pregnancy outcome.

Management

- Those with disability may require extra help during pregnancy and while caring for the infant following delivery.
- There is no contraindication to epidural anaesthesia, except that careful documentation of pre-existing neurological deficit in the legs is necessary to avoid any postpartum exacerbation of MS being inappropriately attributed to the regional block.

Multiple sclerosis – points to remember

- Pregnancy has no effect on the long-term prognosis of MS.
- Attacks are less likely during pregnancy but more likely in the postpartum period.

Myasthenia gravis

Incidence

The prevalence is between 1 in 10 000 and 1 in 50 000 with a female to male preponderance of 2:1.

Clinical features

There may be exacerbations and remissions. The symptoms and signs include the following:

- Diplopia
- Ptosis
- Dysphagia
- Respiratory muscle weakness (in severe cases).

Pathogenesis

Myasthenia gravis is caused by IgG antibodies directed against the nicotinic acetylcholine receptor on the motor endplate. These block neuromuscular transmission at the postsynaptic level, causing weakness and fatigue of skeletal, but not smooth muscle.

Diagnosis

- The diagnosis is made by administration of edrophonium chloride, a short-acting anticholinesterase. This produces prompt but transient improvement in muscle strength (the Tensilon test).
- Electromyography typically shows a reduction in evoked muscle potential following repetitive, supramaximal muscle motor-nerve stimulation.
- Acetylcholine receptor antibodies are found in up to 90% of patients and an associated thymoma in 10%.

Pregnancy

Effect of pregnancy on myasthenia gravis

- In approximately 40% of women, pregnancy is associated with exacerbation of the disease. In 30%, there is no change; in 30%, remissions occur.
- Exacerbation in pregnancy is less likely if the woman has undergone previous thymectomy.
- The course of myasthenia gravis is not necessarily the same in different pregnancies in the same woman.

▪ Postpartum exacerbations occur in 30% of women.

▪ The physiology of pregnancy may also indirectly influence the disease. For example, nausea and vomiting in early pregnancy, delayed gastric emptying and gastrointestinal absorption, and increased volume of distribution and renal clearance, may all lead to subtherapeutic levels of medication.

Effect of myasthenia gravis on pregnancy

▪ There is a high incidence of preterm delivery and growth restriction (40%).

▪ Since the uterus has smooth muscle, the first stage of labour is unaffected by myasthenia; however, maternal effort using voluntary striated muscle is required in the second stage, and this may be impaired.

Neonatal myasthenia gravis

▪ Up to 20% of neonates born to myasthenic mothers may be affected by neonatal myasthenia due to transplacental passage of IgG antibodies. This usually becomes apparent in the first 2 days after birth, and is characterised by difficulty in feeding, crying, a floppy baby and respiratory embarrassment.

▪ It is transient, resolves within 2 months, corresponding to the disappearance of maternal antibodies in the neonate, and responds to anticholinesterase drugs.

▪ The delayed onset of neonatal myasthenia contrasts with congenital heart block (see chapter 8, p. 145) caused by transplacental passage of anti-Ro antibodies, which usually affects the fetus *in utero*. The explanation may be:
  – Transfer of maternal drugs across the placenta
  – Differences between fetal and adult acetylcholine receptors
  – An inhibitory effect of the α-fetoprotein in amniotic fluid on the binding of antibody to the acetylcholine receptor.

▪ There is no way to predict which neonates will be affected but it is related to the titre of acetylcholine receptor antibodies.

Management

▪ Most patients with myasthenia gravis are treated with the long-acting anticholinesterase, pyridostigmine; this drug should be continued in pregnancy.

▪ Increased doses may be required as pregnancy advances; this may be more appropriately achieved by decreasing the dosage interval rather than increasing each dose.

▪ In large doses, these drugs may cause nausea, vomiting, diarrhoea and hypersalivation, and overdose can result in paradoxical weakness and respiratory failure.

▪ A vaginal delivery should be the aim, although instrumental delivery may be required to prevent the woman from becoming exhausted. Caesarean section should only be performed for the usual obstetric indications.

- Anticholinesterase drugs should be given parenterally in labour to avoid erratic absorption due to delayed gastric emptying.
- Some patients respond to corticosteroids and these should be maintained in pregnancy.
- Azathioprine and plasmapheresis (for crises) have also been used.
- Thymectomy is also employed in the treatment of myasthenia gravis, but its use is not recommended in pregnancy.

Other drugs and women with myasthenia gravis

- Consultation with an experienced obstetric anaesthetist is advisable, preferably prior to delivery.
- Epidural analgesia and anaesthesia are safe to use but the ester type of local anaesthetics (e.g. chlorprocaine, tetracaine) depend on maternal plasma cholinesterase for their metabolism, and should be avoided if the mother is being treated with anticholinesterases.
- Lignocaine and the amide type of local anaesthetics are metabolised by a different pathway and are therefore safe for use in labour and delivery.
- If an inhalational anaesthetic is required, ether and halothane should be avoided.
- Myasthenics are also particularly sensitive to non-depolarising muscle relaxants such as curare and suxamethonium, which may have an exaggerated or prolonged effect.
- Other drugs that may exacerbate or cause muscle fatigue include aminoglycosides (gentamicin), β-adrenergics (ritodrine, salbutamol) and narcotics.
- Although magnesium sulphate is the drug of choice for seizure prophylaxis in eclampsia and pre-eclampsia (see chapter 1), it should be avoided in women with myasthenia gravis since it may precipitate a crisis.

Myasthenia gravis – points to remember

- The course of myasthenia gravis in pregnancy is unpredictable.
- Postpartum exacerbations occur in 30% of women.
- Increased doses of long-acting anticholinesterases may be required as pregnancy advances.
- Many drugs should be avoided in myasthenia gravis and consultation with an experienced obstetric anaesthetist is recommended.
- Up to 20% of neonates born to myasthenic mothers may be affected by neonatal myasthenia due to transplacental passage of IgG antibodies.

Incidence

Myotonic dystrophy is a rare degenerative neuromuscular and neuroendocrine disease. Pregnancy in severely affected women is rare. In some milder cases, the disease may only be recognised in pregnancy.

Clinical features

This is an autosomal dominant inherited disorder. The characteristic features include:

- Progressive muscular dystrophy
- Muscle weakness
- Myotonia (failure to relax after forceful contraction)
- Myopathic facies (due to weakness of facial muscles)
- Cataracts
- Frontal alopecia
- Mental retardation
- Heart conduction defects
- Pneumonia and hypoventilation.

Pregnancy

Effect of pregnancy on myotonic dystrophy

- Pregnancy may be associated with marked exacerbations of myotonia and muscle weakness, or symptoms may be unchanged.
- Deterioration may occur early in pregnancy but is most severe in the third trimester.
- Improvement after delivery is rapid.

Effect of myotonic dystrophy on pregnancy

- There is an increased risk of:
  - First and second trimester miscarriage
  - Stillbirth
  - Polyhydramnios (indicative of an affected fetus)
  - Premature delivery (also more common with an affected fetus)
  - Placenta praevia.
- The second trimester losses and premature delivery may be related to abnormal myotonic involvement of the uterus.
- Abnormalities of all three stages of labour have been described. Both pro-

172

longed and rapid first and second stages are reported. Uterine inertia responds to oxytocin.

■ Postpartum haemorrhage is common due to failure of uterine contractions in the third stage.

■ The baby may be affected with congenital myotonic dystrophy, which is distinct from the adult form and probably arises from a combination of the autosomal dominant gene and an intrauterine environmental factor. The disease is rare with an affected father.

■ The congenital syndrome includes:
  – Severe generalised hypotonia and weakness
  – Difficulties in breathing, sucking and swallowing
  – Talipes
  – Arthrogryposis
  – Mental retardation.

Myotonia and cataracts are usually absent.

Management

■ Prenatal diagnosis is possible by direct DNA analysis from chorion villus biopsy.

■ General anaesthesia should be avoided and great care is needed with respiratory depressants such as opiates that may exacerbate pulmonary hypoventilation.

■ Referral to an obstetric anaesthetist is recommended.

Benign intracranial hypertension (BIH)

Incidence

This condition is commonest in obese, young women.

Clinical features

■ Headache, often retro-orbital
■ Obesity, rapid weight gain
■ Diplopia
■ Papilloedema
■ Cerebrospinal fluid (CSF) pressure is increased.

Diagnosis

The combination of papilloedema and raised intracranial pressure without CT or MRI evidence of hydrocephalus or a space-occupying lesion.

Pregnancy

Effect of pregnancy on BIH

- BIH may present for the first time in pregnancy, commonly in the second trimester.
- Pre-existing BIH tends to worsen during pregnancy, possibly related to weight gain.

Management

- Limitation of weight gain.
- Monitor visual fields and visual acuity. In severe cases, infarction of the optic nerve may occur, leading to blindness. Any impairment of visual acuity or in the visual fields should prompt treatment with corticosteroids.
- Repeated CSF drainage or insertion of a shunt may provide relief from headache.
- Thiazide diuretics may reduce intracranial pressure and may be continued throughout pregnancy if required.

Stroke

The risks of arterial ischaemic stroke, cerebral venous thrombosis, and intracranial haemorrhage are increased, particularly in the puerperium.

Ischaemic stroke

Incidence

- Strokes are rare in women of child-bearing age (3.5 in 100 000).
- Pregnancy increases the risk of cerebral infarction (5–200 in 100 000), but this risk is largely due to a nine-fold increased risk during the puerperium.
- Patients who have had stroke in the past may be reassured that they are very unlikely to have recurrence in pregnancy unless they have an obvious risk factor such as antiphospholipid syndrome (see chapter 8, p. 146).

Clinical features

- Most strokes associated with pregnancy occur in the distribution of the carotid and middle cerebral arteries.
- Most cases occur in the first week after delivery.

Pathogenesis

- The risk factors of hypertension, smoking and diabetes for stroke in non-pregnant patients are found less commonly in pregnancy-associated strokes.

- Cerebral infarction may rarely occur following classical migraine.
- Unusual causes of strokes are more common in pregnancy, such as:
  - Mitral valve prolapse
  - Peripartum cardiomyopathy (see chapter 2, p. 32)
  - Antiphospholipid syndrome (see chapter 8, p. 146)
  - Vasculitis (SLE, Takayasu's disease)
  - Subacute bacterial endocarditis (SBE)
  - Sickle-cell disease
  - Thrombotic thrombocytopenic purpura (TTP)
  - Paradoxical embolus (in situations causing increased right compared with left atrial pressure)
  - Pre-eclampsia/eclampsia (see chapter 1, p. 7).

Diagnosis

- MRI or CT is appropriate to confirm ischaemic stroke and differentiate haemorrhage from infarction.
- Investigations to establish a cause should include echocardiography.

Management

- This depends on the underlying cause.
- It is safe to continue or start low-dose aspirin in pregnancy.
- Anticoagulation may be appropriate.

Intracerebral haemorrhage

Incidence

- This is very rare in women of child-bearing age (where there is a preponderance of cerebral infarction as a cause of stroke) outside pregnancy, but is almost as common as ischaemic stroke in pregnancy.
- The relative risk in pregnancy is 2.5 and during the puerperium 28.
- There were nine deaths in the UK due to intracerebral haemorrhage in the 1994–1996 Confidential Enquiry into maternal deaths.

Pathogenesis

- Eclampsia. Intraparenchymal haemorrhage is found in 40% of women dying from eclampsia. The haemorrhage is thought to be due to cerebral vasospasm, loss of autoregulatory control and breakthrough of the vessel wall (see chapter 1, p. 8).

- Ruptured vascular malformations. Whether pregnancy increases the risk of rupture of arteriovenous malformations (AVMs) is controversial. The rate of first cerebral haemorrhage is not increased by pregnancy and the risk of a second haemorrhage is not known accurately.
- AVMs are oestrogen sensitive and therefore tend to dilate in pregnancy.
- Reported haemorrhages from AVMs occur fairly evenly throughout gestation and the postpartum period. About 6% occur during labour and delivery.

Management

- If an AVM is diagnosed pre-pregnancy, pregnancy should be deferred until after treatment.
- AVMs may not be amenable to surgery. There are no data concerning embolisation of AVMs in pregnancy. Stereotactic radiotherapy is not used in pregnancy because it exposes the fetus to large amounts of gamma irradiation.
- In women with untreated AVMs, there is no advantage of caesarean over vaginal delivery and the former should be reserved for the usual obstetric indications.

Subarachnoid haemorrhage (SAH)

Incidence

- 20 in 100 000 pregnancies.
- The risk of SAH is increased two- to three-fold during pregnancy and 20-fold in the puerperium.
- Bleeding from either an aneurysm or an AVM is associated with a high rate of maternal morbidity and mortality.
- There were 15 deaths due to SAH in the UK between 1994 and 1996.

Clinical features

- Headache (sudden and severe, often occipital)
- Vomiting
- Loss of or impaired consciousness
- Sudden collapse
- Neck stiffness
- Papilloedema
- Focal neurological signs are often, but not invariably present.

Pathogenesis

- SAH may be due to a ruptured arterial (berry) aneurysm or to AVM.

- Outside pregnancy, the ratio of aneurysm to AVM is 7:1.
- In pregnancy, relatively more cases are due to AVMs. The ratio is 1:1.
- The classic notion that rupture of an arterial aneurysm occurs more frequently during labour, related to Valsalva manoeuvres, has not been confirmed.
- In one study of ruptured aneurysms related to pregnancy, 90% occurred antenatally, 8% during the puerperium and only 2% during labour and delivery.
- The risk of bleeding from arterial aneurysms increases progressively with successive trimesters.
- This suggests haemodynamic, hormonal or other physiological changes of pregnancy may play a role in aneurysm rupture.

Diagnosis

- CT or MRI will confirm the diagnosis and determine the site of the bleed.
- Magnetic resonance angiography is used to identify the cause of the bleeding.
- Angiography should not be withheld because of the pregnancy.

Management

- Neurosurgical management for SAH should not differ from that of the non-pregnant woman.
- There is neurosurgical consensus to treat asymptomatic aneurysms >7–10 mm.
- Clipping of aneurysms has been successful during all stages of pregnancy.
- Surgical management is associated with lower maternal and fetal mortality rates.
- The risk of re-bleeding from an AVM in the remainder of pregnancy may be as high as 50%.
- If the AVM or aneurysm is successfully operated upon, then vaginal delivery is preferable.
- If the lesion has not been operated on, elective caesarean section does not improve maternal or fetal outcome. It may be appropriate if there has been acute bleeding near term or for fetal salvage if the mother is moribund.
- Measures to decrease the risk of recurrent bleeding during vaginal delivery include epidural anaesthesia (which is also recommended to avoid the hypertensive response to intubation of the trachea, in the event of an emergency caesarean section), and a short second stage with possible low instrumental delivery.
- Regional anaesthesia is contraindicated in cases of recent SAH, when there is a risk of raised intracranial pressure.

■ If epidural block is not used, β-adrenergic blockade will attenuate a hypertensive response to intubation.

Bell's palsy

Incidence

■ This condition occurs much more commonly in pregnancy (10-fold increase).
■ Incidence is approximately 45 in 100 000 pregnancies.

Clinical features

■ There is a unilateral lower motor neurone lesion of the facial (VIIth cranial) nerve.
■ This causes facial weakness, including loss of frontalis muscle (the patient cannot wrinkle her forehead) on the affected side.
■ There may be associated pain around the ear or loss of taste on the anterior two-thirds of the tongue.
■ Most cases in pregnancy occur around term, either in the 2 weeks before or after delivery.

Pathogenesis

■ The lesion is due to swelling of the facial nerve within the petrous temporal bone, but the underlying cause is not known. The reason for the increased incidence in late pregnancy may be related to oedema.
■ Ramsay Hunt syndrome is herpes zoster (shingles) of the geniculate ganglion and causes a unilateral facial palsy (identical to Bell's) with herpetic vesicles in the external auditory meatus and occasionally the soft palate.
■ Very rarely, Bell's palsy may be bilateral, in which case the differential diagnosis should include:
  – Guillain–Barré syndrome
  – Sarcoidosis
  – Lyme disease.

Diagnosis

The diagnosis is made on clinical grounds.

Management

■ Bell's palsy usually improves spontaneously (90%), but this may happen slowly over a period of months.

- There is no evidence that pregnancy-associated Bell's palsy is associated with a worse outcome.

- A short (2-week) course of corticosteroids (prednisolone 40 mg/day, tapered after the first week) may speed recovery, but this needs to be instituted as soon as possible (preferably within 24 hours after the onset of symptoms).

- Steroids should not be given in Ramsay Hunt syndrome and therefore it is imperative to examine the ear for vesicles prior to the prescription of corticosteroids.

Cerebral vein thrombosis

The reader should consult Chapter 3, p. 57.

Further reading

Crawford, P., Appleton, R., Betts, T. et al. (1999) Best practice guidelines for the management of women with epilepsy. *Seizure*, **8**, 201–217.

Grosset, D.G., Ebrahim, S., Bone, I. and Warlow, C. (1995) Stroke in pregnancy and the puerperium: what magnitude of risk? *J. Neurol. Neurosurg. Psychiatr.*, **58**, 129–131.

Hudspith, M.J. and Popham, P.A. (1986) The anaesthetic management of intracranial haemorrhage from arteriovenous malformations during pregnancy: three cases. *Int. J. Obstet. Anaesth.*, **5**, 189–193.

Jaffe, R., Mock, M., Abramowicz, J. and Ben-Aderet, N. (1986) Myotonic dystrophy and pregnancy: a review. *Obstet. Gynecol. Surv.*, **41**, 272–278.

Kittner, S.J., Stern, B.J., Feeser, B.R. et al. (1996) Pregnancy and the risk of stroke. *N. Engl. J. Med.*, **335**, 768–774.

Mas, J-L. and Lamy, C. (1998) Stroke in pregnancy and the puerperium. *J. Neurol.*, **245**, 305–313.

Pfaffenrath, V. (1998) Migraine in pregnancy: what are the safest treatment options? *Drug Safety*, **19**, 383–388.

Plauche, W.C. (1983) Myasthenia gravis. *Clin. Obstet. Gynecol.*, **26**, 592–604.

Rudnik-Schoneborn, S., Nicholson, G.A., Morgan, G., Rorig, D. and Zerres, K. (1998) Different patterns of obstetric complications in myotonic dystrophy in relation to the disease status of the fetus. *Am. J. Med. Genet.*, **80**, 314–321.

CHAPTER 10
Renal disease

Physiological adaptation	Specific types of renal disease
Urinary tract infection	Pregnancy in dialysis patients
Chronic renal disease	Renal transplant recipients
	Acute renal failure

Physiological adaptation

(Table 10.1)

■ There is a dramatic dilatation of the urinary collecting system during pregnancy. This may be the result of ureteral smooth-muscle relaxation induced by progesterone, or a compression of the ureters by the enlarging uterus or iliac vessels. Caliceal and ureteral dilatation is more pronounced on the right.

Table 10.1 – Physiological renal changes in pregnancy

Physiological variable	Direction of change	Percentage increase or normal range for pregnancy
RPF	↑	60–80%
GFR	↑	55%
Creatinine clearance	↑	120–160 ml/min
Protein excretion	↑	<300 mg/24 hours
Urea	↓	2.0–4.5 mmol/l
Creatinine	↓	25–75 μmol/l
Bicarbonate	↓	18–22 mmol/l
Uric acid	↓	↑ with gestation (see Appendix 2)

GFR: glomerular filtration rate; RPF: renal plasma flow.

- Renal plasma flow (RPF) rises very early in pregnancy and has increased by 60–80% by the second trimester of pregnancy.
- RPF falls throughout the third trimester but is still maintained at 50% greater than pre-pregnancy values at term.
- Glomerular filtration rate (GFR) also increases significantly and creatinine clearance rises by about 50%. This results in a fall in the serum urea and creatinine levels.
- Protein excretion is increased and the upper limit of normal in pregnancy is taken as 300 mg/24 hours.
- There is physiological sodium (and water) retention during pregnancy; 80% of pregnant women develop some oedema, especially towards term, so it is usually not a pathological sign. The pregnant woman has a decreased ability to excrete a sodium and water load and this is most marked near term.

Urinary tract infection

This may be divided into the following:

- Asymptomatic bacteriuria
- Acute cystitis
- Acute pyelonephritis.

Although urinary tract infection (UTI) is a common and important problem in pregnancy, it should never be assumed to be the cause of abdominal pain and/or proteinuria before further investigation to confirm or refute the diagnosis is undertaken.

Asymptomatic bacteriuria

Incidence

- This affects 4–7% of pregnant women, of whom up to 40% will develop symptomatic urinary tract infection in pregnancy. Of pregnant women, 2% develop pyelonephritis.
- Women who have a history of previous urinary tract infection and are found to have bacteriuria have a 10-fold increased risk of developing cystitis or acute pyelonephritis in pregnancy.

Pathogenesis

- 75–90% of bacteriuria in pregnancy is due to *Escherichia coli*, probably derived from the large bowel.
- Colonisation of the urinary tract results from ascending infection from the perineum and is related to sexual intercourse.

Diagnosis

■ Most women with asymptomatic bacteriuria are infected during early pregnancy. Very few subsequently acquire asymptomatic bacteriuria.

■ Bacteriuria is only considered significant if the colony count exceeds 100 000/ml on a mid-stream urine (MSU) specimen.

■ Urine culture resulting in a non-significant or mixed growth should be repeated on a fresh MSU specimen.

■ Dipsticks for nitrites and leucocyte esterase may be used to help exclude UTI.

Management

■ Because dilation of the upper renal tract during pregnancy increases the risk of pyelonephritis (see later), asymptomatic bacteriuria should be treated.

■ Treating asymptomatic bacteriuria reduces the risk of preterm delivery and low birthweight babies.

■ The choice of antibiotic depends on the sensitivities of the causative organism.

■ Ampicillin, amoxycillin, Augmentin and the cephalosporins are safe and appropriate antibiotics for use in pregnancy. Treatment with cefadroxil 500 mg b.d. is effective against the majority of urinary pathogens.

■ Nitrofurantoin 100 mg t.d.s. and trimethoprim 200 mg b.d. are safe alternatives. Nitrofurantoin used in the third trimester may precipitate neonatal haemolytic anaemia. Trimethoprim should be avoided in the first trimester due to its anti-folate action.

■ Long-acting sulphonamides should be avoided in the last few weeks of pregnancy because they increase the risk of neonatal kernicterus. Septrin (co-trimoxazole = trimethoprim + sulphamethoxazole) is no longer recommended for treatment of urinary tract infection.

■ Treatment for 3 days is sufficient for asymptomatic bacteriuria. Regular urine cultures should be taken following treatment to ensure eradication of the organism. About 15% of women will have recurrent bacteriuria during their pregnancy and require a second course of antibiotics.

Acute cystitis

Incidence

Cystitis complicates about 1% of pregnancies.

Clinical features

■ These include urinary frequency, dysuria, haematuria, proteinuria and suprapubic pain.

■ Urinary tract infection in pregnancy is more common in diabetics (both with pre-existing and gestational diabetes) and in those receiving systemic cortico-steroids.

Pathogenesis

See 'Asymptomatic bacteriuria' (earlier). Most infections are due to *E. coli.*

Diagnosis

■ This is confirmed by the finding of significant bacteriuria (see earlier) following culture of a MSU specimen.

■ Microscopy of the urine may reveal organisms, white cells and occasionally red cells, but the false-positive rate is very high and it is no longer recommended for diagnosis of UTI.

Management

■ This is the same as for asymptomatic bacteriuria (see earlier).

■ Antibiotic therapy is guided by sensitivities of the organism. For organisms resistant to penicillins, cephalosporins, nitrofurantoin and trimethoprim; ciprofloxacin may be appropriate but this is not used as first-line therapy in pregnancy.

■ Antibiotics should be continued for 5–7 days.

■ Several non-pharmacological manoeuvres may help prevent recurrent infection in those women troubled by urinary tract infections in pregnancy. These include:
  – Increasing fluid intake. This ensures frequent voiding and a high volume dilute urine, all of which reduce the risk of symptomatic infection.
  – Emptying the bladder following sexual intercourse. This 'washes away' organisms massaged up the urethra from the perineum into the bladder during coitus, before they have a chance to replicate in urine within the bladder.
  – Double voiding (to ensure no residual urine is left in the bladder following micturition).
  – The perineum should be cleaned from 'front to back' following defaecation to minimise the risk of bowel organisms colonising the urethra.

Acute pyelonephritis

Incidence

■ This complicates 1–2% of pregnancies.

■ It is more common in pregnancy because of the physiological dilatation of the upper renal tract.

Clinical features

- These include fever, loin and/or abdominal pain, vomiting, rigors as well as proteinuria, haematuria and concomitant features of cystitis (see earlier).
- Like cystitis, it is more common in women with diabetes and those on steroid therapy.

Other risk factors include:

- Polycystic kidneys
- Congenital abnormalities of the renal tract (for example, duplex kidney or ureter)
- Neuropathic bladder (e.g. in those with spina bifida or multiple sclerosis)
- Urinary tract calculi.

Pathogenesis

See 'Asymptomatic bacteriuria' (earlier). Most infections are due to *E. coli*. Cultures yielding significant growths of mixed organisms should prompt a search for underlying renal calculi.

Diagnosis

- This is confirmed by the finding of significant bacteriuria (see earlier) following culture of a MSU specimen.
- Differential diagnosis includes pneumonia (especially right lower lobe), viral infections, cholecystitis and biliary colic, acute appendicitis, gastroenteritis, placental abruption and a degenerating uterine fibroid (see also Section B, Tables 12 and 17.)
- Investigation in women with fever should include blood cultures and a full blood count.

Pregnancy

- Acute pyelonephritis increases the risk of premature labour at least in part because of associated pyrexia.
- There is also evidence for an increased risk of low birthweight babies, but this is partly related to an increase in preterm delivery.

Management

- This should be undertaken in hospital.
- Once the diagnosis is suspected and a urine sample obtained, antibiotic treatment with appropriate i.v. antibiotics should begin immediately, before awaiting the results of urine culture or sensitivities.

- I.v. penicillins or cephalosporins (e.g. cefuroxime) are usually the first choice, although in the case of septicaemia or resistant organisms or women who are allergic to both penicillins and cephalosporins, an aminoglycoside such as gentamicin may be used. There is a theoretical risk of fetal ototoxicity with the use of gentamicin in pregnancy, but provided drug levels are measured and kept within the therapeutic range, this should not be a problem encountered in clinical practice.
- Antibiotics should be given intravenously until the pyrexia settles, when they may be changed to an appropriate oral formulation. Antibiotics should be continued for a period of at least 2 weeks.
- Renal function should be checked regularly since renal impairment may complicate acute pyelonephritis in pregnancy, especially if there is associated sepsis.
- I.v. fluids may also be required if the woman is volume depleted as a result of vomiting or sweating.
- An ultrasound examination of the kidneys should be undertaken to exclude hydronephrosis, congenital abnormalities and renal calculi.

Prophylaxis

- Women who usually take antibiotic prophylaxis against urinary tract infections should continue this in pregnancy.
- Suitable regimes in pregnancy include low-dose amoxycillin or low-dose oral cephalosporins (cephalexin 250 mg), or nitrofurantoin 50 mg o.d., but depend on the sensitivities of the usual infecting organisms.

Urinary tract infection – points to remember

- Urinary tract infection is more common in pregnancy.
- Asymptomatic bacteriuria should be treated because there is a significant risk of acute pyelonephritis.
- Acute pyelonephritis increases the risk of premature labour.
- Acute pyelonephritis should be managed in hospital with i.v. antibiotics.
- Once antibiotic treatment has rendered the urine sterile, regular MSU specimens are necessary to exclude reinfection.
- Amoxycillin and cephalosporins are appropriate antibiotics for the treatment and prevention of UTI in pregnancy.
- Gentamicin may be required for severe or resistant infections.
- Investigations in cases of pyrexia and suspected acute pyelonephritis should include blood cultures, a full blood count, renal function and a renal US.

■ Once a woman has had two or more confirmed and documented UTIs in pregnancy, renal ultrasound (US) should be performed and antibiotic prophylaxis considered.

Chronic renal disease

Pregnancy

Effect of pregnancy on chronic renal disease

The risks include:

■ Possible accelerated decline in renal function
■ Escalating hypertension during pregnancy
■ Worsening proteinuria during pregnancy.

Increased proteinuria is a physiological response to pregnancy and may not necessarily indicate superimposed pre-eclampsia or deteriorating renal disease.

Effect of chronic renal disease on pregnancy

The risks include:

■ Miscarriage
■ Pre-eclampsia
■ Intrauterine growth restriction (IUGR)
■ Preterm delivery
■ Fetal death.

Factors influencing outcome

The outcome of pregnancy and any adverse effect on underlying renal disease are both influenced by:

■ Presence and degree of renal impairment (see later)
■ Presence and severity of hypertension
■ Presence and degree of proteinuria
■ Underlying type of chronic renal disease (see later).

In general, women without hypertension or renal impairment prior to conception have successful pregnancies and pregnancy does not adversely influence the progression of the renal disease.

Degree of renal impairment

■ Degree of renal impairment is traditionally divided into mild (plasma creatinine <125 μmol/l), moderate (plasma creatinine >125 μmol/l and <250 μmol/l), and severe (plasma creatinine >250 μmol/l).

- Absolute creatinine levels may be misleading if allowance is not made for the size of the woman. For example, a plasma creatinine level of 200 μmol/l in a woman weighing 50 kg represents a greater reduction in renal function than the same level in a woman weighing 80 kg.
- Women with severe renal impairment should be advised against pregnancy.

Effect of pregnancy on renal impairment

- Women with more severe renal impairment are more likely to have an accelerated decline and/or a permanent worsening of renal function as a result of the pregnancy (Table 10.2).

Table 10.2 – Effect of pregnancy on renal impairment

Degree of renal impairment	Mild Cr < 125 μmol/l	Moderate < 170 μmol/l	< 220 μmol/l	Severe Cr > 220 μmol/l
Loss of function	2%	40%	65%	75%
Postpartum deterioration		20%	50%	60%
End-stage renal failure		2%	33%	40%

Cr: creatinine.

- Initially in all but those with very severe renal impairment, the usual increase in GFR occurs, leading to a fall in the serum creatinine level early in pregnancy. However in those with moderate and severe renal impairment, the serum creatinine level usually begins to rise to and beyond pre-pregnancy levels during the second trimester.

Effect of degree of renal impairment on pregnancy outcome

- Women with more severe renal impairment are at increased risk of adverse pregnancy outcome and complications – especially pre-eclampsia, IUGR, and prematurity (Table 10.3).
- Polyhydramnios (and the accompanying risks of preterm rupture of the membranes and cord prolapse) may complicate pregnancies where the maternal urea level is greater than 10 mmol/l. This results from fetal polyuria due to the osmotic load from the high maternal urea level.
- Once the maternal urea level is greater than 20–25 mmol/l, there is a risk of fetal death.

Table 10.3 – Effect of degree of renal impairment on pregnancy outcome

Degree of renal impairment	Mild Cr < 125 μmol/l	Moderate 125–249 μmol/l	Severe Cr > 250 μmol/l
Problems, e.g. pre-eclampsia	25%	50%	85%
IUGR		30%	60%
Preterm		55%	70%
Success	85–95%	60–90%	20–30%

Cr: creatinine.

Specific types of renal disease

Glomerulonephritis

- Most pregnancies are successful. Those with hypertension are at increased risk of superimposed pre-eclampsia.
- Fetal loss and preterm delivery rates are about 20%.
- Less than 10% have a reversible and 3% a progressive decrease in renal function related to pregnancy.
- Over 25% have a reversible and <10% a permanent increase in blood pressure.
- In those with normal renal function at conception, pregnancy does not affect the course of renal disease or the occurrence of end-stage renal failure. Hypertension and proteinuria accelerate the rate of decline in renal function, whether or not a woman has been pregnant.

Reflux nephropathy

- This is one of the most common renal diseases in women of child-bearing age.
- About 25% of women develop pre-eclampsia and this risk is increased in cases of bilateral renal scarring.
- Even those with normal renal function and without hypertension pre-pregnancy are at increased risk of hypertension (33%) and pre-eclampsia (15%).
- Those with renal impairment may experience rapid worsening of renal function.
- There is a particular association between reflux nephropathy in the mother and severe IUGR.
- Reflux nephropathy may be inherited as an autosomal dominant condition, and therefore offspring of affected mothers should be screened with a micturating cystogram, as US may miss the diagnosis.

Diabetic nephropathy (see also chapter 5)

- Adverse pregnancy outcome and maternal complications are doubled compared to pregnant diabetics without nephropathy.
- The specific risks are urinary tract infection, pre-eclampsia, proteinuria and oedema that may be severe but usually revert after delivery to pre-pregnancy levels.
- Nephrotic syndrome can be severe with marked hypoalbuminaemia and the risk of pulmonary oedema and thrombosis.
- Over 30% of affected women have preterm deliveries and over 50% have an increase in blood pressure.
- Most women with diabetic nephropathy show the normal increase in GFR and pregnancy does not increase the rate of deterioration in renal function.

SLE nephritis

(See chapter 8).

Polycystic kidney disease (PKD)

- This is an autosomal dominant disorder usually presenting in the fourth decade with hypertension, recurrent urinary tract infections, haematuria or renal impairment. Some asymptomatic women are aware of their diagnosis because of affected family members and positive screening. Women may remain undiagnosed throughout pregnancy.
- The risks in pregnancy are of pre-eclampsia, which is more common in those with pre-existing hypertension or renal impairment, and urinary tract infections. Loin pain and haematuria may occur without urinary tract infection.
- Pregnancy has no adverse long-term effect on renal function.
- PKD may be associated with polycystic liver disease and subarachnoid haemorrhage from intracranial aneurysms. Liver cysts may enlarge during pregnancy and those with a family history of intracranial aneurysms should be screened for aneurysms prior to pregnancy.
- Since PKD is an autosomal dominant disorder, there is a 50% chance of transmission to the affected woman's offspring.

Management of pregnancies complicated by chronic renal disease

- Management should begin with pre-pregnancy counselling. Assessment of pre-conceptual renal function and blood pressure enables accurate counselling and provides a baseline with which to compare trends in pregnancy.

■ Obstetricians and physicians who have expertise in the care of renal disease in pregnancy should manage jointly women with chronic renal disease.

■ In view of the increased risk of pre-eclampsia, treatment with low-dose aspirin should be considered, especially in those with hypertension and renal impairment or a previous poor obstetric history.

■ Careful monitoring and control of blood pressure both pre-pregnancy and antenatally is important. Treatment for blood pressure problems is no different from the management of pregnant women without renal disease (see chapter 1, p. 12); however the threshold for treatment may be lower, since good control of hypertension is important to preserve renal function.

■ Regular assessment of renal function by creatinine clearance and 24-hour protein excretion, as well as serum creatinine and urea is essential. It may be useful to give the woman urine testing strips so she can monitor the presence and severity of any proteinuria or haematuria.

■ The fetus should be monitored with regular US assessment of growth and Doppler assessment of uterine and umbilical circulation.

■ Admission should be considered if the woman develops worsening hypertension, deteriorating renal function or proteinuria, superimposed pre-eclampsia, or polyhydramnios.

■ As discussed in chapter 8, the differentiation between pre-eclampsia and deterioration of pre-existing renal disease may be extremely difficult. However, the

---

Chronic renal disease – points to remember

■ Women with chronic renal disease are at increased risk of pre-eclampsia, IUGR, preterm delivery and caesarean section; the perinatal mortality rate is increased.

■ These obstetric complications and the risk of permanent deterioration in renal function are increased by the presence and severity of any renal impairment or hypertension.

■ For women with moderate or severe renal impairment (plasma creatinine >125 μmol/l), up to 60% of infants are born prematurely and the risk of acceleration of decline in renal function is 25–50%.

■ An increase in the degree of proteinuria is very common in pregnancy and does not necessarily imply pre-eclampsia or worsening renal disease.

■ Management should include regular monitoring of blood pressure, renal function and fetal well-being.

■ In view of the increased risk of pre-eclampsia, treatment with low-dose aspirin should be considered, especially in those with hypertension and renal impairment or a previous poor obstetric history.

indications for renal biopsy during pregnancy are mostly limited to situations where a delay before delivery is desirable (i.e. before 32 weeks' gestation) and a diagnosis of a steroid or chemotherapy-sensitive lesion is suspected.

Pregnancy in dialysis patients

- Fertility is reduced in women on haemodialysis or chronic ambulatory peritoneal dialysis (CAPD). The pregnancy rate is about 1 in 200 women per year.
- The chance of successful pregnancy outcome is low (30%) with both haemodialysis and CAPD.
- Poor prognostic features for pregnancy in dialysis patients include:
  - Age >35 years
  - More than 5 years on dialysis
  - Delayed diagnosis of pregnancy (leading to late increase in dialysis times).

Effect of pregnancy on renal replacement therapy

- Anaemia is exacerbated by pregnancy. Transfusion requirements increase. Erythropoietin and i.v. iron may be safely used and increased in pregnancy.
- Pregnancy is associated with markedly increased requirements for dialysis.
- Doses of heparin may need to be increased to prevent clotting of dialysis lines.
- Pregnancy causes fluctuations in fluid balance and blood pressure.
- Doses of vitamin D and calcium may need to be reduced.

Effect of dialysis on pregnancy

- The risks include:
  - Miscarriage
  - Intrauterine death
  - Hypertension and pre-eclampsia
  - Preterm labour
  - Preterm rupture of membranes
  - Polyhydramnios related to uraemia
  - Placental abruption.
- Full heparinisation requirements during haemodialysis increase the risk of bleeding.
- The specific problems with CAPD include peritonitis.

Management

- In women on haemodialysis, the duration and/or the frequency of dialysis must be increased, to more than 20 hours/week.
- The aim should be to maintain the pre-dialysis urea at less than 15–20 mmol/l.

■ Dietary restrictions can usually be lifted, although continued adherence to fluid restriction is important to avoid large fluid shifts during dialysis.

Renal transplant recipients

■ Women receiving renal transplants should be warned that as renal function returns to normal, ovulation, menstruation and fertility also resume.

■ Women desiring pregnancy are usually advised to wait about 1–2 years after transplantation, by which time graft function has stabilised and maintenance levels of immunosuppressive drugs will have been reached, thus minimising any risk to the fetus.

■ Survival is improved for recipients of living, related donors compared to cadaveric donors.

■ Successful pregnancy outcome for those transplant recipients who become pregnant and do not miscarry before 12 weeks is now 95%.

■ As with chronic renal impairment, pregnancy outcome and effects on the renal allograft are both dependent on the baseline serum creatinine level and the presence of hypertension; the poorer the graft function at conception, the higher the risk of complications and deterioration in graft function.

Pregnancy

Effect of pregnancy on renal transplants

■ Pregnancy has no adverse long-term effect on renal allograft function or survival in women with baseline creatinine levels of <100 μmol/l.

■ For women who enter pregnancy with a serum creatinine level >130 μmol/l, renal graft survival is only 65% at 3 years.

■ Renal allografts adapt to pregnancy in the same way as normal kidneys, and exhibit an increase in GFR and collecting-system dilatation. As with normal kidneys, the GFR may decrease again in the third trimester.

■ About 15% of women develop significant impairment of renal function during pregnancy and this may persist after delivery.

■ About 40% of women develop proteinuria towards term, but this usually regresses postpartum.

■ More than 10% of women are likely to develop new long-term problems following pregnancy, although whether this is as a direct result of pregnancy is difficult to ascertain. The risk of long-term problems is higher in women developing pregnancy complications prior to 28 weeks' gestation.

■ About 10% of women will die within 1–7 years after pregnancy, and about 50% within 15 years.

Effect of renal transplants on pregnancy

- Outcome is optimal in those without hypertension, proteinuria, recent episodes of graft rejection, and in those with normal or near-normal renal function (serum creatinine level <125 μmol/l).
- The chance of successful outcome beyond 12 weeks is 97% with a baseline creatinine level <125 μmol/l, but this is reduced to 75% if the baseline creatinine level is >125 μmol/l.
- The complication rate is higher for diabetics, and those with poor graft function.
- The incidence of problems in pregnancy is about 50% and includes:
  - Hypertension/pre-eclampsia (30%)
  - Graft rejection (10%)
  - IUGR (20–40%)
  - Preterm delivery (45–60%)
  - Infection, especially urinary tract infection.

Antenatal management

- Women should be managed jointly by nephrologists and obstetricians with expertise in the care of pregnant renal transplant recipients.
- Careful monitoring and control of blood pressure is important.
- Regular assessment of renal function by creatinine clearance and 24-hour protein excretion, as well as serum creatinine and urea is essential.
- A full blood count and liver function tests should also be checked regularly. Anaemia is common and haematinics should be prescribed. Maternal hypocalcaemia and hypercalcaemia are both potential problems, and calcium status should be carefully monitored. Doses of calcium and vitamin D may need to be altered in pregnancy.
- An MSU specimen should be taken and sent at each visit and any infection treated promptly. Some women require prophylactic antibiotics.
- Cytomegalovirus (CMV) titres should be checked in each trimester if the woman is CMV negative at the onset of pregnancy.
- The fetus should be monitored with regular US assessment of growth and Doppler assessment of uterine and umbilical circulation.
- Provided proteinuria is not accompanied by deteriorating renal function or hypertension, this is not an indication for delivery.
- The differential diagnosis of deteriorating renal function includes:
  - Reversible causes, e.g. infection (e.g. urinary tract infection), dehydration
  - Pre-eclampsia
  - Cyclosporin nephrotoxicity
  - Acute and/or chronic rejection.

- The features of acute rejection include:
  - Deteriorating renal function
  - Fever
  - Oliguria
  - Graft swelling and tenderness
  - Altered echogenicity of renal parenchyma and blurring of corticomedullary junction on ultrasound.
- Definitive diagnosis of rejection is only possible with renal biopsy.

Immunosuppressive therapy

- The levels of immunosuppressive drugs are maintained at pre-pregnancy levels. Regimes vary but include treatment with:
  - Prednisolone
  - Azathioprine
  - Cyclosporin
  - Tacrolimus
- Mycophenolate mofetil; this is contraindicated in pregnancy and effective contraception is required during and for 6 weeks after discontinuation of treatment.
- Women require reassurance regarding the relative safety of their drugs, as reduction or cessation of immunosuppressive therapy may provoke rejection.
- Side-effects of prednisolone and azathioprine are discussed in chapters 4 (p. 63) and 8 (p. 138), respectively.
- Azathioprine dose may be monitored via maternal white-cell count.
- Both cyclosporin and tacrolimus appear to be safe for use in pregnancy. Plasma levels should be measured regularly.
- Mycophenolate mofetil (MMF) is teratogenic and women desiring pregnancy should be converted to azathioprine prior to conception. They should be counselled regarding possible detrimental effects on graft function from such a change in therapy. In some cases discontinuation of MMF, and therefore pregnancy, is contraindicated.
- Pregnancy success rates are similar in women taking azathioprine and cyclosporin, but the incidence of IUGR is higher (30–40% versus 20%) in women taking cyclosporin.

Delivery

- Caesarean section is only required for obstetric indications, although the overall section rate is increased (25%) compared to background rates. The renal allograft does not obstruct vaginal delivery.
- Prophylactic antibiotics should be given to cover any surgical procedure, including episiotomy.

■ Parenteral steroids are necessary to cover labour, as with any woman on maintenance steroids (see chapter 4, p. 65).

Neonatal problems

These are largely related to prematurity but also include the following:

■ Thymic atrophy

■ Transient leukopenia or thrombocytopenia

■ Depressed haemopoiesis

■ Adrenocortical insufficiency

■ Septicaemia

■ CMV and hepatitis B infection.

Congenital abnormalities are no more common in the offspring of mothers taking antirejection doses of the earlier mentioned immunosuppressive drugs.

Renal transplants – points to remember

■ If graft function is normal, pregnancy outcome is excellent and there is no adverse long-term effect on renal allograft function or survival.

■ The chance of successful pregnancy outcome is reduced and the risk of long-term deterioration in graft function increased with poor baseline graft function.

■ Pregnancy outcome is optimal in those without hypertension, proteinuria, or recent episodes of graft rejection.

■ The doses of immunosuppressive drugs are maintained at pre-pregnancy levels.

■ Prednisolone, azathioprine, cyclosporin and tacrolimus are safe for use in pregnancy. Mycophenolate mofetil is contraindicated.

■ The risks of pre-eclampsia, graft rejection, IUGR, preterm delivery and infection are increased.

■ Caesarean section is only required for obstetric indications, but the rate is increased.

■ Prophylactic antibiotics should be given to cover any surgical procedure.

Acute renal failure (ARF)

Incidence

■ Acute renal failure is rare in pregnancy ($<0.005\%$), but mild-to-moderate transient renal impairment is more common.

- In the developing world, acute renal failure in pregnancy remains a common cause of maternal mortality.
- In the developed world, renal impairment is much less dangerous than iatrogenic fluid overload, particularly in the context of pre-eclampsia.

Clinical features

- Anuria is unusual and should prompt a search for urinary retention or a blocked urinary catheter.
- Oliguria, especially intra- and postpartum is common and does not indicate acute renal failure unless there is rising urea and creatinine.
- Urea may rise in isolation following corticosteroid administration; this does not indicate ARF.
- The serum sodium level is low; there may be hyperkalaemia and a metabolic acidosis.
- Oliguria may be followed by a period of polyuria.
- There may be evidence of pre-existing renal impairment.

Pathogenesis (see also Section B, Table 13)

The causes of acute renal failure in pregnancy include the following:

- *Infection*: septic abortion, puerperal sepsis, rarely acute pyelonephritis.
- *Blood loss*: postpartum haemorrhage, abruption.
- *Volume contraction*: pre-eclampsia, eclampsia (6%), hyperemesis gravidarum.
- *Post-renal failure*: ureteric damage or obstruction.
- *Drugs*: non-steroidal anti-inflammatory drugs (NSAIDs), antibiotics.

In many of these situations, there is an associated coagulopathy. The constellation of acute renal failure, microangiopathic haemolytic anaemia and thrombocytopenia may be due to the following:

- Pre-eclampsia (see chapter 1).
- Haemolysis, Elevated Liver enzymes, and Low Platelets (HELLP) syndrome (7% have acute renal failure) (see chapter 11, p. 212).
- Thrombotic thrombocytopenic purpura (TTP)/haemolytic uraemic syndrome (HUS) (see chapter 14, p. 266).
- Acute fatty liver of pregnancy (AFLP) (see chapter 11, p. 209).

The commonest cause of ARF in the context of pre-eclampsia is HELLP syndrome (about 50%).

Diagnosis

- The underlying cause of ARF may be obvious, for example in the case of abruption and postpartum haemorrhage, although abruption occurs in 16% of women with HELLP syndrome and this may be the true underlying cause.
- Blood loss may not be recognised or may be underestimated, and the diagnosis only made upon the finding of a low CVP. Hypotension may be absent or masked by co-existent pre-eclampsia.
- The differentiation between pre-renal (volume depletion or blood loss) and renal (acute tubular or cortical necrosis) causes is important, since the treatment of each is different.
- Often ARF is seen postpartum, where there are features of pre-eclampsia with thrombocytopenia, and differentiation of HELLP syndrome from HUS may be difficult.
- Pointers to HELLP syndrome, which is far more common, are abnormal liver function, a coaguloapthy (not seen in HUS) and a lower grade haemolysis.
- Pointers to HUS are profound thrombocytopenia, and florid microangiopathic haemolytic anaemia.

Management

- This depends on the underlying cause, but in all cases accurate assessment of fluid balance with a urinary catheter and central venous pressure (CVP) line is essential. Measurements of fluid input and output should be made hourly.
- The treatment of pre-renal failure is adequate replacement of blood and fluid losses. Diuretics should be avoided until volume depletion has been corrected.
- Any associated coagulopathy must be treated (see chapter 14, p. 264).
- Once volume depletion has been excluded or treated, fluids are infused at a rate of 20 ml/hour (to allow for insensible losses) plus the volume of the previous hour's urine output. This can be averaged out over 24 hours to allow for i.v. drug administration and equates to about 500 ml plus the total output of the previous day.
- Fluid overload must be prevented, especially in pre-eclampsia, because of the susceptibility of these women to pulmonary oedema (see chapter 1, p. 17).
- There is no place for 'fluid challenges' in the context of a high or normal CVP.
- Acute tubular necrosis is reversible and supportive management is continued until recovery is apparent.
- Plasmapheresis is not needed for HELLP syndrome, which usually improves with conservative therapy.
- Dialysis may become necessary in ARF to prevent or treat uraemia, acidosis,

hyperkalaemia or fluid overload, but a requirement for long-term renal replacement therapy is very unusual.

Further reading

Armenti, V.T., Ahlswede, K.M., Ahlswede, B.A. et al. (1995) Variables affecting birth weight and graft survival in 197 pregnancies in cyclosporin treated female kidney transplant recipients. *Transplantation,* **59,** 476.

Cattell, W.R. (1997) Urinary tract infection in women. *J. Roy. Coll. Physic. Lond.,* **31,** 130–133.

Davison, J. and Baylis, C. (1995) Renal disease. In: de Swiet, M. (ed.) *Medical Disorders in Obstetric Practice,* 3rd edn, Oxford: Blackwell Science. pp 226–305.

Epstein, F.H. (1996) Pregnancy and renal disease. *N. Engl. J. Med.,* **335,** 277–278.

Hou, S.H. (1999) Pregnancy in women with chronic renal insufficiency and end stage renal disease. *Am. J. Kid. Dis.,* **33,** 235–252.

Jones, D.C. and Hayslett, J.P. (1996) Outcome of pregnancy in women with moderate or severe renal insufficiency. *N. Engl. J. Med.,* **335,** 226–232.

Jungers, P., Houllier, P., Forget, D. et al. (1995) Influence of pregnancy on the course of primary chronic glomerulonephritis. *Lancet,* **346,** 1122–1124.

Jungers, P. and Chauveau, D. (1997) Pregnancy in renal disease. *Kidney Int.,* **52,** 871–885.

Smaill, F. (1999) Antibiotics for asymptomatic bacteriuria in pregnancy (Cochrane review). In: The Cochrane Library. Issue 1. Oxford: update software.

CHAPTER 11

Liver disease

Physiological changes	Obstetric cholestasis
Hyperemesis gravidarum	Acute fatty liver of pregnancy
Viral hepatitis	HELLP syndrome
Pre-existing liver disease	

Physiological changes

■ Pregnancy is associated with increased liver metabolism.

■ The total serum protein concentration decreases, largely because of the 20–40% fall in serum albumin concentration. Some of this decrease may be explained by dilution due to the increase in total blood volume.

■ Concentrations of fibrinogen are dramatically increased, and there are rises in the concentrations of caeruloplasmin, transferrin and many of the specific binding proteins such as thyroid-binding globulin (TBG) and corticosteroid-binding globulin (CBG).

■ There is no significant change in bilirubin concentration during normal pregnancy, but the alkaline phosphatase concentration increases dramatically two- to four-fold. This is largely due to placental production, which increases with successive trimesters. The upper limit of normal for alkaline phosphatase increases from about 130 U/l in the first trimester to over 400 U/l in the third trimester.

■ There is a fall in the upper limit of the normal ranges for both alanine transaminase (ALT), serum glutamic pyruvic transaminase (SGPT) and aspartamine transaminase (AST), serum glutamic-oxaloacetic transaminase (SGOT) throughout pregnancy from about 40 U/l in the first trimester to below 30 U/l in the third. The concentrations of other liver enzymes are not substantially altered. (See table of normal ranges, Appendix 2).

Hyperemesis gravidarum

(see also chapter 12)

Hyperemesis with severe or protracted vomiting in early pregnancy, sufficient to cause fluid, electrolyte and nutritional disturbance, may be associated with abnormal liver function tests in up to 50% of cases. The most usual abnormalities are:

- A moderate rise in transaminases (50–200 U/l)
- Slightly raised bilirubin (jaundice is uncommon).

Hyperemesis is a diagnosis of exclusion (see 'Differential diagnosis of abnormal liver function tests' in Section B, Table 15).

- Associated epigastric pain should raise the possibility of peptic ulcer, pancreatitis or cholecystitis.
- Significant elevation of transaminases, especially in the presence of jaundice, should prompt a search for viral hepatitis.

As the hyperemesis improves spontaneously or is treated (see chapter 12), the abnormalities in liver function resolve.

Viral hepatitis

Worldwide, viral hepatitis is the commonest cause of hepatic dysfunction in pregnancy. Causes include:

- Hepatitis viruses A, B, C, D or E (Table 11.1)
- Cytomegalovirus (CMV)
- Epstein–Barr virus (EBV)
- Herpes simplex virus (HSV).

With the important exception of hepatitis E and herpes simplex infection, the clinical features of viral hepatitis in the pregnant woman do not differ from those in the non-pregnant woman.

Hepatitis A

This is caused by a virus transmitted via the faecal–oral route, and is an acute, self-limited illness that does not result in chronic infection. Maternal–fetal transmission is rare but may result if the mother develops hepatitis A at or around the time of delivery. In such cases, the neonate should be given immune globulin at birth.

Hepatitis B (HBV)

- 170 million people are chronically infected with hepatitis B worldwide. The prevalence in developed countries is about 0.2%. Carriage among pregnant women in the UK is 0.1–0.5% but up to 1% in inner city areas.
- The risk of perinatal infection from asymptomatic mothers is high, and greatest for mothers who are both hepatitis B surface-antigen (HBsAg) positive and hepatitis B e-antigen (HbeAg) positive (vertical transmission 95%).

Table 11.1 – Viral hepatitis in pregnancy

Virus	Transmission	Vertical transmission	Timing of maternal infection giving maximum risk to fetus/neonate	Treatment to protect neonate
Hepatitis A	Faecal–oral	Rare	Near delivery	Immune globulin at birth
Hepatitis B	Blood	Common (especially if HbeAg positive)	Puerperium (i.e. infectious at delivery)	Hepatitis B Ig Hepatitis B vaccine
Hepatitis C	Blood	Uncommon	Third trimester	
Hepatitis D	Blood	Uncommon		Hepatitis B Ig Hepatitis B vaccine
Hepatitis E	Faecal–oral	? Common	? Near delivery	

■ Women who are HBsAg positive, but HbeAg negative have a 2–15% vertical transmission risk. Measurement of viral DNA has replaced e-antigen as the most sensitive test of viral activity.

■ Treatment of hepatitis B is possible with interferon-α or lamivudine. Response rates to interferon are about 40%.

■ Maternal–neonatal transmission usually occurs at delivery, but may also be transplacental (5%).

■ Neonates infected at birth have a >90% chance of becoming chronic carriers of HBV with the associated risks of subsequent cirrhosis and hepatocellular carcinoma.

■ All neonates born to women with acute or chronic HBV should be given hepatitis B immune globulin and HBV vaccine within 24 hours of birth. Immunisation is 85–95% effective at preventing both HBV infection and the chronic carrier state.

■ Provided babies are immunised, there is no need to prevent HBsAg-positive mothers from breast-feeding.

Hepatitis C (HCV)

■ Up to 300 million people worldwide have chronic hepatitis C infection. Prevalence in the UK is about 0.3–0.7%.

- Hepatitis C is the primary cause of non-A, non-B hepatitis and the commonest cause of post-transfusion hepatitis (about 85% of patients contracting post-transfusion non-A non-B hepatitis prior to 1991 are HCV-antibody positive).

- However only 15% of those infected in the UK have a history of transfusion of blood or blood products.

- The commonest (75%) risk factor for hepatitis C infection in the UK is past or current i.v. drug use.

- Of i.v. drug users in the UK, 50–90% are HCV infected.

- Sexual transmission is unusual and <5% of long-term sexual partners become infected.

- There is a significant risk (60–80%) of chronic infection. About 20% of those with chronic infection develop slowly progressive cirrhosis over a period of 10–30 years. Detection of HCV antibody implies persistent infection rather than immunity.

- The risk of progressive liver disease is lower in women, those aged <40 years, and those who do not abuse alcohol.

- Interferon-α combined with tribavirin is more effective than α-interferon alone. About 30% of those with viral genotypes 0, 1, or 2 will have a sustained response following 1 year of combination therapy. Of those with viral genotypes 3, 4, or 5 treated for 6 months, 54% will demonstrate a sustained response.

- Side effects of interferon therapy include a fever or flu-like illness in 80%, fatigue in 50%, depression in 25% and haematological abnormalities in 10%. Only 15% of patients receiving interferon therapy experience no side effects.

Pregnancy

- Pregnancy does not induce deterioration in liver disease.

- There is no evidence of increased risk of adverse pregnancy outcome, however women with hepatitis C antibodies have an increased risk of obstetric cholestasis (OC) that may present earlier than usual (see later).

- Viral load is an important risk factor for vertical transmission that occurs predominantly in women positive for HCV RNA as well as anti-HCV antibody (Table 11.2). In women with chronic HCV, maternal ALT levels do not affect rates of transmission.

- Co-infection with human immunodeficiency virus (HIV) is a major risk factor for vertical transmission of HCV.

- In the neonate, hepatitis C virus (HCV) infection can only be reliably detected using the polymerase chain reaction to detect HCV RNA, as all infants of HCV-antibody-positive mothers will have detectable levels of maternal HCV antibody for the first few months of life.

Table 11.2 – Vertical transmission rate for HBV, HCV and HIV related to the serostatus of the mother

Infection	Serostatus of mother		Vertical transmission rate (%)
HBV	HB$_s$Ag+	HBeAg– and HBV DNA–	2–15
	HB$_s$Ag+	HBeAg+ and HBV DNA+	80–95
HCV	HCV Ab+	HCV RNA–	<1
	HCV Ab+	HCV RNA+	11
	HCV Ab+	HCV RNA+ and HIV Ab+	16
HIV	HIV Ab+		15–20

Hepatitis B surface antigen (HbsAg), hepatitis B virus DNA (HBV DNA), hepatitis B e-antigen (HBeAg), hepatitis C virus antibodies (HCV Ab), hepatitis C virus RNA (HCV RNA), HIV antibodies (HIV Ab), negative (−), positive (+).

- There are no vaccines to prevent HCV infection. Immune globulin is not recommended for infants of HCV-positive mothers.
- Transmission by breast milk is uncommon.

Hepatitis delta virus (HDV)

This virus is only found in HBsAg-positive people, most of whom are HbeAg negative. Prevention of HBV infection or transmission will also prevent HDV infection.

Hepatitis E (HEV)

- This is the enteric form of non-A, non-B hepatitis.
- It has caused several epidemics in association with contaminated water in developing countries. Outbreaks have been reported in India, Ethiopia, Mexico and the Middle East.
- It causes a mild, self-limiting disease, similar to hepatitis A virus infection, in the non-pregnant woman.
- There is a dramatically increased mortality rate in pregnant women, particularly if the virus is acquired in the third trimester. There is an increased incidence of hepatic encephalopathy and fulminant hepatic failure.
- The risk of fulminant hepatic failure with acute hepatitis E infection in pregnancy is 15%, with a mortality rate of 5%.
- The virus has a predilection for pregnant women; the reason for this is not known.

Herpes simplex virus (HSV)

■ This is rare but may cause fulminant hepatitis in the pregnant woman, with an associated high mortality rate.

■ Most cases are due to primary HSV type 2 infections, although oral or vulval vesicles may only appear after presentation with liver failure.

■ Clinical features include fever and abdominal pain. Jaundice is unusual, but there is usually marked elevation in the transaminases, and there may be prolongation of the prothrombin time.

■ Since the infection is usually disseminated, patients may have associated pneumonitis or encephalitis.

■ Diagnosis is made on liver biopsy, which shows extensive focal haemorrhagic necrosis and intranuclear inclusion bodies adjacent to the necrotic areas. Electron microscopy may reveal viral particles and the biopsy can also be stained with HSV antibodies. Viral culture of the liver biopsy, and serology detecting IgG and IgM HSV antibodies may be helpful.

■ Disseminated HSV should be treated with i.v. antiviral therapy. Acyclovir therapy for the infant can also be used to prevent transmission.

Obstetric cholestasis (OC)

Obstetric cholestasis is a disease unique to pregnancy. The exact incidence is not known, but it is more prevalent in certain populations, particularly those of Scandinavia, Chile (incidence up to 12%), Bolivia and China. The prevalence in European countries is about 1%, although women of Indian and Pakistani descent seem to have a higher risk.

Clinical features

■ Severe pruritus affecting the limbs and trunk, particularly the palms and soles, developing in the second half of pregnancy (usually during the third trimester).

■ Associated insomnia and malaise are common.

■ There may be excoriations, but no rash.

■ Liver function tests are abnormal.

■ There may be associated dark urine, anorexia, and malabsorption of fat with steatorrhoea.

■ If OC develops in HCV antibody-positive women, onset of symptoms is earlier in gestation (mean 29 weeks) than HCV antibody-negative women (mean 34 weeks).

■ Complete recovery is usually rapid following delivery, although rarely the condition may worsen postpartum. In some women, abnormal liver function tests may return to normal only slowly, taking 4–6 weeks to reach normal values.

Pathogenesis

The pathogenesis is not clearly understood, but appears to relate to a predisposition to the cholestatic effect of increased circulating oestrogens, and progestogens may also play a role.

Genetic factors

- Positive family history may be found in about 35% of patients.
- Family studies suggest autosomal dominant sex-limited inheritance.

Oestrogen

- Exogenous oestrogens (combined oral contraceptive pill) may precipitate a similar syndrome.
- Elevated oestrogens are associated with significant impairment in sulphation capacity (sulphation of bile acids is important in attenuating their cholestatic potential).

A decrease in hepatocyte membrane fluidity is also implicated, possibly correlated with a defect in the methylation of membrane phospholipids and a modification in the cholesterol:phospholipid ratio.

Diagnosis

OC is a diagnosis of exclusion. The diagnosis is therefore made in three steps:

- A typical history of pruritus without rash
- Abnormal liver function tests
- Exclusion of other causes of itching and abnormal liver function.

The usual pattern of abnormal liver function tests is as follows:

- Moderate (less than three-fold) elevation in transaminases (ALT is the most sensitive)
- Raised alkaline phosphatase (beyond normal pregnancy values)
- Raised gamma-glutamyl transpeptidase (γGT) (about 20% of cases)
- Mild elevation in bilirubin (less common)
- Increased serum total bile acid concentration
- Primary bile acids (cholic acid and chenodeoxycholic acid) may increase 10- to 100-fold
- In some instances, an increased concentration of bile acids may be the only biochemical abnormality
- Pruritus may precede the derangement of liver function tests and serial measurements are advised in women with persistent typical itching.

To exclude other common causes of pruritus and abnormal liver function, the following investigations are recommended:

- Liver ultrasound (the presence of gallstones without evidence of extra-hepatic obstruction does not exclude a diagnosis of OC)
- Viral serology (for hepatitis A, B, and C, EBV, CMV)
- Liver autoantibodies (for pre-existing liver disease; anti-smooth muscle antibody/chronic active hepatitis; anti-mitochondrial antibodies/primary biliary cirrhosis).

The differential diagnoses of pruritus and jaundice in pregnancy are discussed in Section B, Tables 14 and 15, pp 305, 306.

Pregnancy

Maternal risks

- Vitamin K deficiency (malabsorption of fat-soluble vitamins)
- Increased risk of postpartum haemorrhage.

Fetal considerations

- Intrapartum fetal distress (abnormal intrapartum fetal heart rate, e.g. fetal bradycardia, tachycardia or decelerations) (12–22%)
- Amniotic fluid meconium (25–45%)
- Spontaneous preterm delivery (12–44%)
- Intrauterine fetal death
- Fetal intracranial haemorrhage.

The exact magnitude of these risks is difficult to determine, especially as current management protocols include early delivery before the perceived maximum time of risk for the fetus. Thus, reported perinatal mortality rates have fallen from 11% in earlier studies to 2–3.5% in more recent series in which women were delivered before 38 weeks' gestation. Further considerations include:

- The mechanisms whereby OC may adversely affect the fetus are not known.
- The risk of stillbirth increases towards term, but does not correlate with maternal symptoms or transaminase levels.
- The fetal risk may be related to the serum concentration of maternal bile acids:
  - High concentrations of bile acids have been found in amniotic fluid and fetal circulation.
  - Bile acids, especially cholic acid, cause a dose-dependent vasoconstrictive effect on isolated human placental chorionic veins. An abrupt reduction of oxygenated blood flow at the placental chorionic surface leading to fetal asphyxia may be an explanation of fetal distress and demise.
  - Bile acids are toxic to rat cardiac myocytes.

Prediction of fetal compromise

- This remains the most difficult aspect in the management of OC.
- No effect has been demonstrated on the Doppler blood-flow analysis in the uterine, umbilical or fetal cerebral arteries, even in severe cases of OC with high levels of bile acids.
- Repeated amniocentesis to detect meconium may offer the best predictor of fetal compromise.

Management

- Once a diagnosis of OC is made, the affected woman should be counselled concerning the possible risks to the fetus and the need for close surveillance.
- Liver function tests including prothrombin time, and if available, bile acids, should be checked regularly.
- Fetal well-being should be monitored at frequent intervals. Most centres use a combination of cardiotocography (CTG), ultrasound scans for fetal growth and liquor volume and umbilical artery Doppler blood-flow analyses.
- Active management with intense fetal surveillance and early delivery at 37–38 weeks, or when fetal lung maturity is evident, may decrease perinatal mortality.

Drug therapy

Vitamin K

- Vitamin K (10 mg orally, daily) given to the mother may reduce the risk of maternal and fetal bleeding.
- Vitamin K is mandatory for women with a prolonged prothrombin time or receiving concomitant cholestyramine therapy.
- It is preferable to use a water-soluble formulation in view of the often co-existent fat malabsorption.
- Vitamin K therapy is commenced at 32 weeks or from diagnosis (if after 32 weeks) in view of the increased incidence of preterm labour.

Antihistamines
Chlorpheniramine (Piriton®) 4 mg t.d.s. or promethazine (Phenergan®) 25 mg at night may help relieve pruritus.

Ursodeoxycholic acid (UDCA)

- UDCA is an endogenous hydrophilic bile acid that acts by altering the bile acid pool, and reducing the proportion of hydrophobic, and therefore hepatotoxic, bile acids.
- It is a choleretic agent that reduces serum bile acids.

- It has been used extensively outwith pregnancy in other conditions associated with bile salt retention, such as primary biliary cirrhosis.
- Doses of 1000–1500 mg daily in two to three divided doses lead to impressive relief or improvement of pruritus and reduction of total bile acid and liver enzyme levels in most patients.
- UDCA is not licensed for use in pregnancy, but there are no reports of adverse fetal or maternal effects.
- There is no evidence to support or refute a beneficial effect of UDCA on the risk of fetal compromise and death.

Dexamethasone

Dexamethasone suppresses fetoplacental oestrogen production. Given in one study at doses of 12 mg orally, daily, it relieved pruritus and lowered bile acids and transaminases.

Cholestyramine

Questran®, given at a dose of 4 g two to three times daily, is a bile acid-chelating agent that may relieve itching in some women, but is poorly tolerated because it is so unpalatable and may cause gastrointestinal upset. Questran increases the risk of vitamin K deficiency.

S-adenosylmethionine (sAME)

sAME therapy given intravenously may restore normal hepatocyte membrane fluidity. It has improved pruritus and liver biochemistry in some but not all studies.

Activated charcoal

This lowers total bile acid concentrations but has no effect on pruritus.

Epomediol

This may reduce pruritus.

Intrapartum management

- In women who do not deliver prematurely, labour is usually induced at 37–38 weeks' gestation.
- Because of the high risk of fetal distress, close monitoring is required throughout induction and labour.
- The neonate should receive i.m. vitamin K.

Recurrence risk/pre-pregnancy counselling

- Risk of developing OC in future pregnancies is about 90%.

- Women who have had OC should avoid oestrogen-containing oral contraceptives. If they are used, liver function should be monitored.
- Hormone replacement therapy need not be avoided, as this provides only physiological levels of oestrogen.

Obstetric cholestasis – points to remember

- Pruritus in the third trimester should prompt a request for liver function tests.
- The most usual abnormality is elevated transaminases, which may only be mild.
- Frank jaundice is rare now.
- There is a significant risk to the fetus, which is difficult to predict and not mirrored by maternal symptoms.
- Management should focus on relief of maternal symptoms, regular close fetal surveillance, and elective early delivery before 38 weeks' gestation.
- Vitamin K should be given to the mother and neonate.
- The risk of recurrence in future pregnancies is about 90%.
- Women who have had OC should be advised to avoid oral contraceptives containing oestrogen.

Acute fatty liver of pregnancy (AFLP)

Acute fatty liver of pregnancy is rare (1 in 9000 to 1 in 13 000 pregnancies), but potentially lethal for both the mother and fetus, especially if diagnosis is delayed. It is considered by some to be a variant of pre-eclampsia. AFLP is commoner in primigravidae (although this predilection is not as marked as in pre-eclampsia). There is an association with obesity, male fetuses (ratio 3:1) and multiple pregnancy. The high maternal and fetal mortality rate may be lower than originally believed (85%) as milder cases are recognised and appropriately treated. More recent studies suggest figures around 10–20% for maternal mortality and 20–30% for perinatal mortality.

Clinical features

- Usually presents after 30 weeks' gestation, and often near term, with gradual onset of nausea, anorexia and malaise.
- Severe vomiting and abdominal pain should alert the clinician to the diagnosis.

■ There are often co-existing features of mild pre-eclampsia, but hypertension and proteinuria are usually mild.

■ Jaundice usually appears within 2 weeks of the onset of symptoms and there may be ascites.

■ Liver function is abnormal and there is a variable (three- to 10-fold) elevation in transaminase levels and raised alkaline phosphatase.

■ Coagulopathy due to disseminated intravascular coagulation (DIC) may be severe and is often the presenting feature postpartum.

■ There may be associated renal impairment.

■ The woman may develop fulminant liver failure with hepatic encephalopathy.

■ There may be polyuria and features of diabetes insipidus (DI), and the association of transient DI and AFLP is well described (see chapter 7, p. 120).

Pathogenesis

■ AFLP may be a variant of pre-eclampsia.

■ A subgroup of women with AFLP and Haemolysis, Elevated Liver enzymes and Low Platelets (HELLP) syndrome are heterozygous for long chain 3-hydroxy-acyl-coenzyme A dehydrogenase (LCHAD) deficiency, a disorder of mitochondrial fatty acid oxidation. These women may succumb to AFLP or HELLP syndrome when the fetus is homozygous for β-fatty acid oxidation disorders.

■ The mechanism of hepatocellular damage may involve the affected fetus producing abnormal fatty acid metabolites.

Diagnosis

Differential diagnosis from HELLP syndrome is shown in Table 11.3.

Two distinctive features of AFLP that may help in its distinction from HELLP syndrome, are:

■ Profound hypoglycaemia (not invariably present)

■ Marked hyperuricaemia (which is out of proportion to the other features of pre-eclampsia).

Radiological evaluation with magnetic resonance imaging (MRI), computerised tomography (CT) or ultrasound may sometimes show hepatic steatosis, but the liver may appear normal. CT may show decreased attenuation suggestive of fatty infiltration.

Liver biopsy with special stains for fatty change or electron microscopy has been considered the gold standard for diagnosis. The characteristic histopathological lesion is microvesicular fatty infiltration (steatosis) of hepatocytes most prominent in the central zone, with periportal sparing but little or no inflammation or hepatocellular necrosis. Liver biopsy is not always necessary or practical in the presence of coagulopathy.

Table 11.3 – Differential diagnosis of HELLP syndrome and AFLP

Symptom	HELLP	AFLP
Epigastric pain	+	+
Hypertension	+ +	+
Proteinuria	+ +	+
Elevated liver enzymes	+	+ +
Hypoglycaemia	±	+ +
Hyperuricaemia	+	+ +
DIC	+	+ +
Thrombocytopenia (without DIC)	+ +	±
White blood count ↑	+	+ +
Ultrasound/CT	Normal/hepatic haematoma	See text
Multiple pregnancy		+
Primiparous	+ +	+
Male fetus	50%	70% (M:F = 3:1)

Management

■ The optimal management of AFLP involves expeditious delivery and this practice has led to improved prognosis for mother and baby.

■ Severely ill patients require a multidisciplinary team in an intensive care setting.

■ Coagulopathy and hypoglycaemia should be treated aggressively before delivery. Large amounts of 50% glucose may be needed to correct the hypoglycaemia, and fresh frozen plasma and albumin should be given as necessary.

■ Plasmapheresis has been used in some cases.

■ Multiple system failure may necessitate ventilation and dialysis.

■ Patients with fulminant hepatic failure and encephalopathy should be referred to a specialist liver unit. Orthotopic liver transplantation should be considered in patients with fulminant hepatic failure and those who manifest signs of irreversible liver failure despite delivery of the fetus and aggressive supportive care.

Prompt reversal of the clinical and laboratory findings usually follows delivery and may be very dramatic, however significant morbidity is common and often related to severe coagulopathy and the need for repeated operations to control postpartum haemorrhage. If the woman survives the initial episode, a complete recovery without long-term liver damage is the norm.

Recurrence

There are limited data but recurrence has been described and liver function should be closely monitored in subsequent pregnancies. Recurrence is particularly likely in women who are heterozygous for disorders for β-fatty acid oxidation, so screening for LCHAD deficiency may be indicated.

Acute fatty liver of pregnancy – points to remember

- This condition is rare, but potentially fatal.
- The diagnosis should be considered, especially if there is severe vomiting and abdominal pain.
- Differential diagnosis is from HELLP syndrome.
- Liver dysfunction is usually marked with hypoglycaemia, hyperuricaemia, renal impairment and coagulopathy.
- The woman is at risk of fulminant hepatic failure and encephalopathy and may require transfer to a regional liver unit.
- Delivery of the fetus is the correct treatment once hypoglycaemia, coagulopathy and hypertension have been controlled.

HELLP syndrome

- HELLP syndrome is one of several possible crises that may develop as a variant of severe pre-eclampsia (see chapter 1, p. 7).
- The incidence in pre-eclamptic pregnancies is about 5–20%, although many more women with pre-eclampsia, perhaps 20–50%, have mild abnormalities of hepatic enzymes without full-blown HELLP syndrome.
- There is increased maternal (1%) and perinatal mortality (reported rates vary from about 10–60%).

Clinical features

- Epigastric or right upper quadrant pain (65%)
- Nausea and vomiting (35%)
- Tenderness in the right upper quadrant

- Hypertension with or without proteinuria
- Other features of pre-eclampsia
- Acute renal failure (7%)
- Placental abruption (16%). This may be the presenting feature and should always prompt investigation for HELLP syndrome or pre-eclampsia as underlying causes
- Metabolic acidosis.

Pathogenesis

- See under 'Pre-eclampsia' (chapter 1, p. 9).
- The pathogenesis of HELLP syndrome involves endothelial cell injury, micro-angiopathic platelet activation and consumption.
- Differential diagnosis includes AFLP (see earlier and Table 11.3) and haemolytic uraemic syndrome (HUS)/thrombotic thrombocytopenic purpura (TTP)(see p. 266). These conditions (AFLP, HELLP, HUS, TTP, pre-eclampsia) may all form part of a spectrum of endothelial disease.

Diagnosis

- Low-grade haemolysis evident on peripheral blood smear, rarely enough to cause severe anaemia
- Low (usually $<100 \times 10^9/1$) or falling platelets
- Elevated transaminases
- Elevated lactate dehydrogenase (LDH) (indicative of haemolysis)
- Raised bilirubin (unconjugated, reflecting the extent of haemolysis).

The platelet count may fall below $30 \times 10^9/1$ in severe cases and some women develop DIC (20%).

Ultrasound may be useful to exclude hepatic haematoma or other causes of acute upper abdominal pain, for example cholecystitis.

Liver biopsy is rarely performed in this syndrome, and therefore reports of the histological changes are sparse. Most reports describe changes similar to patients with pre-eclampsia and liver involvement but without HELLP. There is fibrin deposition in the periportal regions and along the hepatic sinusoids, and peri-portal haemorrhage. Unlike AFLP, there may be hepatic cell necrosis and sub-capsular haemorrhages.

Differential diagnosis from TTP and HUS is important since delivery rather than plasmapheresis is the optimal management for HELLP syndrome. Remember the following:

- TTP and HUS are both rare compared to HELLP syndrome.
- Abnormal liver function and coagulopathy suggest HELLP rather than TTP, even in the presence of frank haemolysis.

- Co-existence of renal failure is well recognised in HELLP syndrome and does not necessarily imply a diagnosis of HUS.
- Profound thrombocytopenia ($<10 \times 10^9/l$) is unusual in pre-eclampsia and HELLP syndrome.

Effect of HELLP syndrome on pregnancy

Factors contributing to maternal morbidity and mortality include:

- Abruption
- Subcapsular liver haematoma
- Acute renal failure
- Massive hepatic necrosis
- Liver rupture.

Management

- Prompt delivery, especially if there is severe right upper quadrant pain and tenderness, since this is usually the result of liver capsule distension.
- As with all cases of pre-eclampsia, it is important to ensure adequate control of blood pressure prior to delivery.
- Platelet transfusion should be reserved for active bleeding or prior to surgery if the platelet count is below $50 \times 10^9/l$.
- Fresh frozen plasma (FFP) should be given to correct any coagulopathy.
- Corticosteroids given to induce fetal lung maturity have been shown to significantly improve both haematological and hepatic abnormalities in HELLP syndrome.
- Attempting to prolong the pregnancy beyond 24 hours with the use of corticosteroids is not standard management in the UK, but could be considered to avoid extreme prematurity. Such a strategy requires intensive monitoring to ensure the continued safety of the mother.

Postpartum course

- Since delivery is usually expedited in diagnosed cases, a woman may deteriorate before she improves after delivery, developing a very low platelet count, severe hypertension and proteinuria.
- Up to 30% of cases arise postpartum, in women thought to have no or uncomplicated pre-eclampsia. These women are at particularly high risk of pulmonary oedema and renal failure. Management in such cases should be supportive, with strict adherence to fluid management protocols to avoid iatrogenic pulmonary oedema, and control of the blood pressure.

■ Recovery from HELLP syndrome is usually rapid and complete with no hepatic sequelae. The liver enzymes often recover before the thrombocytopenia, although as in other cases of pre-eclampsia, antihypertensives may be required temporarily postpartum.

Recurrence

In future pregnancies, women who have had HELLP syndrome are at a substantially increased risk of developing pre-eclampsia, preterm delivery and intrauterine growth restriction. The risk of recurrent HELLP syndrome, on the other hand, is low (3–5%). For women with essential hypertension that predates the pregnancy complicated by HELLP syndrome, the risk of pre-eclampsia in subsequent pregnancies may be as high as 75%.

HELLP syndrome – points to remember

■ This is one of the potential 'crises' that may develop in pre-eclampsia.

■ Other features of pre-eclampsia such as hypertension may be only mild.

■ The typical features are right upper quadrant pain, nausea and vomiting.

■ There is a risk of DIC, abruption, liver haematoma and liver rupture.

■ Delivery of the fetus is the correct treatment once any hypertension has been controlled.

■ Women may present or deteriorate postpartum and renal impairment is not uncommon.

■ Women are at a greatly increased risk of developing pre-eclampsia in future pregnancies.

■ The risk of recurrent HELLP syndrome is low.

Pre-existing liver disease

Autoimmune chronic active hepatitis (CAH)

Mild treated disease is unlikely to cause problems in pregnancy. The issues relate to immunosuppessive drug regimens (see chapter 8, p. 138), which should be continued in pregnancy to prevent relapse.

Primary biliary cirrhosis (PBC)

This condition usually presents with pruritus and is associated with a raised alkaline phosphatase and γGT. Diagnosis is confirmed by the finding of anti-mitochondrial antibodies. Reported pregnancy outcomes are variable although stable, non-advanced disease is unlikely to cause problems. Pruritus may worsen in pregnancy.

Sclerosing cholangitis (SC)

This is a rare chronic, fibrosing, inflammatory disorder of unknown aetiology affecting the biliary tree. It is associated with inflammatory bowel disease, although the severities of the two conditions are not related. In the only reported series of pregnancies in women with SC, pregnancy outcome was good. The only serious complication was severe pruritus.

Cirrhosis

- Severe hepatic impairment is associated with infertility.
- Liver disease may decompensate during pregnancy and pregnancy should be discouraged in women with severe impairment of hepatic function.
- Bleeding from oesophageal varices is a risk in women with portal hypertension, especially in the second and third trimesters.
- Those with portal hypertension stabilised on propranolol should be advised not to discontinue this in pregnancy since the risks to mother and fetus from variceal bleeding far outweigh any risk of β-blocker therapy in pregnancy.

Liver transplants

- Fertility may return to normal after transplantation.
- Pregnancy should be postponed for 18 months to a year after transplantation to allow stabilisation of function and reduction to maintenance levels of immunosuppressive drugs.
- Immunosuppression must be continued and carefully monitored in specialist units throughout pregnancy. Tacrolimus is not associated with teratogenesis.
- Pregnancy in liver transplant recipients is associated with an increased risk of premature delivery.

Further reading

Girling, J.C., Dow, E. and Smith, J.H. (1997) Liver function tests in pre-eclampsia: importance of comparison with a reference range derived for normal pregnancy. *Br. J. Obstet. Gynaecol.*, **104**, 246–250.

Janczewska, I., Olsson, R., Hultcrantz, R. and Broome, U. (1996) Pregnancy in patients with primary sclerosing cholangitis. *Liver*, **16**, 326–330.

Locatelli, A., Roncaglia, N., Arreghini, A. et al. (1999) Hepatitis C virus infection is associated with a higher incidence of cholestasis of pregnancy. *Br. J. Obstet. Gynaecol.*, **106**, 498–500.

Kennedy, S., Hall, P.M., Seymour, A.E. and Hague, W.M. (1994) Transient diabetes insipidus and acute fatty liver of pregnancy. *Br. J. Obstet. Gynaecol.*, **101,** 387–391.

Palma, J., Reyes, H., Ribalta, J. et al. (1997) Ursodeoxycholic acid in the treatment of cholestasis of pregnancy: a randomized, double-blind study controlled with placebo. *J. Hepatol.*, **27,** 1022–1028.

Raine-Fenning, N. and Kilby, M. (1997) Obstetric cholestasis. *Fetal Mat. Med. Rev.*, **9,** 1–17.

Ryder, S.D. and Beckingham, I.J. (2001) Chronic viral hepatitis. In: ABC of disease of liver, pancreas, and biliary system. *Br. Med. J.*, **322,** 219–221.

Sibai, B.M., Ramadan, M.K., Usta, I., Salama, M., Mercer, B.M. and Friedman, S.A. (1993) Maternal morbidity and mortality in 442 pregnancies with hemolysis, elevated liver enzymes, and low platelets (HELLP syndrome). *Am. J. Obstet. Gynecol.*, **169,** 1000–1006.

Tompkins, J., Thiagarajah, S. (1999) HELLP (hemolysis, elevated liver enzymes, and low platelet count) syndrome: the benefit of corticosteroids. *Am. J. Obstet. Gynecol.*, **181,** 304–309.

CHAPTER 12

Gastrointestinal disease

Physiological changes	Inflammatory bowel disease
Hyperemesis gravidarum	Irritable bowel syndrome
Constipation	Abdominal pain
Reflux oesophagitis	Appendicitis
Peptic ulcer disease	Gall bladder disease
	Pancreatitis

Physiological changes

- Changes in gastrointestinal motility during pregnancy include decreased lower oesophageal pressure, decreased gastric peristalsis and delayed gastric emptying.
- Gastrointestinal motility is inhibited generally during pregnancy, with increased small- and large-bowel transit times.
- These changes may in part be responsible for the common symptoms of constipation and nausea and vomiting in early pregnancy.

Hyperemesis gravidarum

Incidence

- Nausea and vomiting are both common in pregnancy, affecting at least 50% of pregnant women.
- Hyperemesis gravidarum occurs in 0.1–1% of pregnancies.

Clinical features

- Onset is always in the first trimester, usually weeks 6–8.
- Persistent vomiting and severe nausea progress to hyperemesis when the woman is unable to maintain adequate hydration, and fluid and electrolyte as well as nutritional status are jeopardised.
- There is weight loss and ketosis and there may be muscle wasting.

- In addition to nausea and vomiting, there may be ptyalism (inability to swallow saliva) and associated spitting.
- There are usually signs of dehydration with postural hypotension and tachycardia.

Investigations

These usually reveal the following:

- Hyponatraemia
- Hypokalaemia
- Low serum urea
- Metabolic hypochloraemic alkalosis
- Ketonuria
- Raised haematocrit level and increased specific gravity of the urine.
- Abnormal liver function tests (found in up to 50% of cases – see chapter 11, p. 199)
- Abnormal thyroid function tests.

These may be a feature in two-thirds of patients with hyperemesis.

The picture is that of a biochemical hyperthyroidism with a raised free thyroxine and/or a suppressed thyroid-stimulating hormone (TSH).

Patients with these abnormalities are clinically euthyroid without thyroid antibodies, except in the very rare case of thyrotoxicosis presenting in early pregnancy.

The abnormal thyroid function tests do not require treatment and resolve as the hyperemesis improves.

There is an increased incidence of gestational thyrotoxicosis demonstrated in Asians compared to Europeans.

Pathogenesis

- The pathophysiology of hyperemesis is poorly understood. Various hormonal, mechanical and psychological factors have been implicated.
- There is a direct relationship between the severity of hyperemesis and the degree of biochemical hyperthyroidism, and it has been suggested that the raised thyroxine levels or suppressed TSH may be causative.
- The level of human chorionic gonadotropin (hCG), which shares a common α-subunit with TSH, is directly correlated with the severity of vomiting and free thyroxine concentrations, and inversely correlated with TSH levels. hCG probably acts as a thyroid stimulator in patients with hyperemesis. There is structural homology not only in the hCG and TSH molecules but also in their receptors, and this suggests the basis for the reactivity of hCG with the TSH receptor.

- The positive correlation between severity of hyperemesis and hCG levels explains the increased incidence of this condition in multiple pregnancy and hydatidiform mole. The theory is also supported by the fact that the peak in hCG levels (in weeks 6–12) coincides with the presentation of hyperemesis.
- Other hormonal deficiencies or excesses, involving follicle-stimulating hormone (FSH), progesterone, cortisol and adrenocorticotrophic hormone (ACTH), have been proposed as aetiological factors, but never proven.
- The physiological changes in oesophageal pressure, gastric peristalsis and gastric emptying may well exacerbate the symptoms of hyperemesis, but are unlikely to be causative in isolation.
- Many psychological and behavioural theories have been suggested to explain hyperemesis, usually involving hyperemesis as an expression of rejection of the pregnancy. Although there is often a psychological component to the condition, it is very difficult to prove causation since hyperemesis itself may cause extreme psychological morbidity. This relates to separation from family, inability to work, anger that the woman feels at being neither blooming nor even well, and guilt when this anger is turned inwards towards the fetus and resentment of the pregnancy results.
- Certainly psychological factors do play a role in a proportion of cases and this may be evident by the rapid improvement on admission to hospital and consequent removal from a stressful home environment.

Diagnosis

- Hyperemesis is a diagnosis of exclusion.
- There is no single confirmatory test.
- Vomiting beginning after week 12 of amenorrhoea should not be attributed to hyperemesis.
- Other causes of nausea and vomiting must be considered, most commonly urinary tract infection, and more rarely Addison's disease (insidious onset with some features predating the pregnancy), peptic ulceration or pancreatitis (abdominal pain is not a prominent symptom in hyperemesis).
- Hyperemesis tends to recur in subsequent pregnancies, so a previous history makes the diagnosis more likely.

Effect of hyperemesis on pregnancy

Maternal complications

- There were three deaths in the Confidential Enquiry into Maternal Deaths in the UK (1991–1993). Two deaths were probably the result of Wernicke's encephalopathy (see later) and one the result of aspiration of vomitus.

- Serious morbidity and mortality may result if hyperemesis is inadequately or inappropriately treated.

Wernicke's encephalopathy

Wernicke's encephalopathy due to vitamin B_1 (thiamine) deficiency is characterised by diplopia, abnormal ocular movements, ataxia and confusion. The typical ocular signs are a sixth nerve palsy, gaze palsy or nystagmus.

- Wernicke's encephalopathy may be precipitated by i.v. fluids containing dextrose.
- There is an increased incidence of abnormal liver function tests in women with hyperemesis complicated by Wernicke's encephalopathy compared to the incidence in hyperemesis in general. As in alcoholics, the abnormal functioning liver may participate in the development of Wernicke's encephalopathy by decreased conversion of thiamine to its active metabolite thiamine pyrophosphate and by a decreased capacity to store thiamine.
- Diagnosis of Wernicke's encephalopathy may be confirmed by the finding of a low red cell transketolase (thiamine-dependent enzyme).
- Enhanced magnetic resonance imaging (MRI) in acute Wernicke's encephalopathy may reveal symmetrical lesions around the aqueduct and fourth ventricle, which resolve after treatment with thiamine.
- Although institution of thiamine replacement may improve the symptoms of Wernicke's encephalopathy, if retrograde amnesia, impaired ability to learn and confabulation (Korsakoff psychosis) have supervened, the recovery rate is only about 50%.

Hyponatraemia

Hyponatraemia (plasma sodium, 120 mmol/l) causes lethargy, seizures and respiratory arrest.

- Both severe hyponatraemia, and particularly its rapid reversal, may precipitate central pontine myelinolysis (osmotic demyelination syndrome). This is associated with symmetrical destruction of myelin at the centre of the basal pons and causes pyramidal tract signs, spastic quadraparesis, pseudobulbar palsy and impaired consciousness.
- Central pontine myelinolysis and Wernicke's encephalopathy may co-exist during pregnancy and thiamine deficiency may render the myelin sheaths of the central pons more sensitive to changes in serum sodium.

Other vitamin deficiencies

Other vitamin deficiencies occur in hyperemesis, including cyanocobalamin (vitamin B_{12}) and pyridoxine (vitamin B_6) causing anaemia and peripheral neuropathy.

Mallory–Weiss tears

Prolonged vomiting may lead to Mallory–Weiss tears of the oesophagus and episodes of haematemesis.

Malnutrition

Protein and calorie malnutrition results in weight loss, which may be profound (10–20%), and muscle wasting with consequent weakness.

Psychology

The psychological problems (see earlier) resulting from severe hyperemesis are often underestimated. Certain problems may pre-date the onset of hyperemesis, but others result from the condition itself. Requests for termination of pregnancy should not be assumed to indicate or confirm that the pregnancy was not wanted, but rather this should be an indication of the degree of desperation felt by the patient.

Total parenteral nutrition

If total parenteral nutrition (TPN) is required, this is usually given via a central venous catheter, and this has its own problems (e.g. infection, pneumothorax).

Thrombosis

Since hyperemesis results in dehydration and is usually associated with bed rest, it constitutes a risk factor for thromboembolism.

Fetal complications

- Wernicke's encephalopathy is associated with a 40% incidence of fetal death.
- Initially it was thought that hyperemesis was not associated with any adverse fetal outcome and there is indeed no increase in the risk of congenital malformations for affected individuals. However, it has been shown that of infants of mothers with severe hyperemesis associated with abnormal biochemistry and weight loss, >5% have significantly lower birthweights and birthweight percentiles compared to infants of mothers with mild hyperemesis and those of the general antenatal population.
- Women admitted repeatedly for hyperemesis have a more severe nutritional disturbance, associated with a significantly reduced maternal weight gain. Infants of women admitted on multiple occasions for hyperemesis have significantly lower birthweights than infants of mothers requiring only a single admission.

Management

- The potential maternal and fetal complications of hyperemesis argue for early and aggressive treatment.

■ Any woman who is ketotic and unable to maintain adequate hydration should be admitted to hospital.

■ An ultrasound scan of the uterus should be performed to confirm gestational age, and to diagnose multiple pregnancy and exclude hydatidiform mole, both of which are associated with an increased incidence of hyperemesis.

I.v. fluid therapy

■ Adequate and appropriate fluid and electrolyte replacement is the most important component of management.

■ Infusion of dextrose-containing fluids (dextrose saline, 5% dextrose, 10% dextrose) is mistakenly thought by some to be desirable to provide the patient with at least some calories, but this assumption is erroneous and dangerous. Firstly, as discussed earlier, Wernicke's encephalopathy may be precipitated by carbohydrate-rich foods or dextrose administered intravenously. Secondly, the hyponatraemia demands the infusion of sodium-containing fluids (dextrose saline contains only 30 mmol/l of Na+ and 5% dextrose contains none).

■ Normal saline (sodium chloride 0.9%; 150 mmol/l Na+) or Hartmann's solution (sodium chloride 0.6%; 131 mmol/l Na+) are appropriate solutions, and potassium chloride is added to the infusion bags as required. There is no place for the use of double-strength saline (2n saline), even in cases of severe hyponatraemia, as this results in too rapid a correction of serum sodium with the risk of central pontine myelinolysis.

■ Fluid and electrolyte regimes must be adapted daily and titrated against daily measurements of serum sodium and potassium and fluid-balance charts.

■ Because of the practical difficulties of maintaining fluid-balance charts over many days in busy wards, the patient should be weighed at least twice weekly to obtain an objective assessment of improvement or deterioration.

Thiamine therapy

■ Thiamine supplementation should be given to anyone suffering from prolonged vomiting. Requirements for thiamine increase during pregnancy to 1.5 mg/day, and women admitted with a diagnosis of hyperemesis have usually been vomiting for at least 1–2 weeks prior to admission. If the woman is able to tolerate tablets, thiamine can be given as thiamine hydrochloride tablets 25–50 mg t.d.s. If i.v. treatment is required for those unable to tolerate tablets, this is given as thiamine 100 mg diluted in 100 ml of normal saline and infused over 30–60 minutes. The i.v. preparation is only required weekly. Treatment (as opposed to prevention) of Wernicke's encephalopathy requires much higher doses of thiamine.

■ Drugs that may cause nausea and vomiting should be temporarily discontinued. The commonest example is iron supplements.

■ All patients with hyperemesis require emotional support with frequent reassurance and encouragement from nursing and medical staff. Psychiatric referral may be appropriate in certain cases.

■ The natural history of hyperemesis is gradual improvement with increasing gestation, although in a minority of women symptoms may persist beyond 20 weeks' gestation.

■ The only definitive cure is termination of the pregnancy.

Pharmacological treatment

Anti-emetics

Anti-emetics should be offered to women failing to respond to i.v. fluids and electrolytes alone.

■ Extensive data exist to show a lack of teratogenesis with:
  – antihistamines (H_1 receptor antagonists, e.g. promethazine, cyclizine)
  – phenothiazines (chlorpromazine, prochlorperazine)
  – dopamine antagonists (metoclopramide, domperidone).

Post-thalidomide anxiety has resulted in an understandable reluctance to prescribe anti-emetics for hyperemesis.

■ Possible regimens include:
  – Cyclizine 50 mg p.o./i.m./i.v. t.d.s.
  – Promethazine 25 mg p.o. nocte
  – Stemetil 5 mg p.o. t.d.s.; 12.5 mg i.m./i.v. t.d.s.
  – Metoclopramide 10 mg p.o./i.m./i.v. t.d.s.
  – Domperidone 10 mg p.o. q.d.s.; 30–60 mg p.r. t.d.s.
  – Chlorpromazine 10–25 mg p.o.; 25 mg i.m. t.d.s.

■ If symptoms do not improve, the anti-emetic should be *prescribed and given regularly* rather than on an 'as required'/p.r.n. basis.

■ Side effects include drowsiness, particularly with the phenothiazines, and extrapyramidal effects and oculogyric crises, particularly with metoclopramide and the phenothiazines.

Ondansetron

■ This highly selective 5-HT_3 (serotonin) antagonist is used with dramatic effect for postoperative and chemotherapy-induced nausea and vomiting.

■ It has been used with success in intractable hyperemesis, but in a comparative study i.v. ondansetron 10 mg was no better than i.v. promethazine 50 mg. However in this study the hyperemesis was not very severe, which may explain the lack of difference in efficacy.

- There is no evidence to support a teratogenic effect of ondansetron but reports of use of this drug are very limited.

Histamine$_2$-receptor blockers

Histamine$_2$-receptor blockers, ranitidine, cimetidine and the proton-pump inhibitor, omeprazole, are used in cases where dyspeptic symptoms accompany the nausea and vomiting of hyperemesis. They appear to be safe for use in pregnancy.

Total parenteral nutrition

- TPN may become necessary supportive therapy in very severe cases of hyperemesis.
- TPN has also been shown to have a rapid therapeutic effect in some cases.
- Metabolic and infectious complications are a risk and strict protocols and careful monitoring are obligatory. The catheter site must be inspected regularly for signs of infection.
- Phlebitis and thrombosis are other recognised complications of TPN. Catheter-related endothelial disruption may provoke thrombosis, but in addition the direct endothelial injury secondary to a hyperosmolar infusate is likely to contribute.
- Because TPN involves the use of high concentrations of glucose, thiamine supplementation is mandatory.
- In addition, parenteral hyperalimentation is expensive and is usually reserved for extremely severe life-threatening cases.
- The author would not recommend TPN for hyperemesis before optimal rehydration and anti-emetic therapy and only after a trial of corticosteroids and/or ondansetron had failed to result in improvement.

Enteral feeding

- When the gastrointestinal tract is intact and usable, it is preferable to use enteral rather than parenteral hyperalimentation to treat malnutrition.
- Enteral hyperalimentation may be poorly tolerated because of nausea and vomiting and may even be contraindicated because of the risk of aspiration.
- Frequent tube displacement may also be a problem. Poor tolerance of a nasogastric tube can be bypassed by use of a gastrostomy feeding tube.
- To minimise the risk of aspiration, the feeding tube may be placed beyond the pylorus, but this necessitates radiation exposure for correct positioning of the tube.
- The cost of enteral feeding is considerably less than that of TPN.

■ The successful use of enteral feeding via a nasogastric tube in hyperemesis unresponsive to anti-emetics has been reported in women with meal-related nausea and vomiting only.

Corticosteroids

■ Corticosteroids have resulted in dramatic and rapid improvement in case series of women with severe refractory hyperemesis. Randomised studies also support a beneficial effect.

■ They should not be used until conventional treatment with i.v. fluid replacement and regular anti-emetics has failed.

■ Suggested doses are prednisolone 40–50 mg p.o. daily in divided doses or hydrocortisone 100 mg i.v. b.d.

■ In cases that do respond to steroid therapy, the dose must be reduced slowly and prednisolone cannot usually be discontinued until the gestation at which the hyperemesis would have resolved spontaneously (in some extreme cases this occurs at delivery).

Pre-pregnancy counselling/recurrence

■ Hyperemesis almost invariably recurs in subsequent pregnancies.

■ In very severe cases, especially those necessitating TPN or termination of the pregnancy, women may be advised that studies suggest a beneficial effect of steroids, which may provide a therapeutic option in subsequent pregnancies.

Hyperemesis gravidarum – points to remember

■ Hyperemesis is a diagnosis of exclusion.

■ Hyperemesis may be associated with both abnormal liver and thyroid function tests.

■ The main risk in hyperemesis is from Wernicke's encephalopathy, resulting from thiamine deficiency.

■ Adequate and appropriate (normal saline) fluid and electrolyte replacement is the most important component of management.

■ Thiamine supplementation should be given to all women admitted with hyperemesis.

■ The common anti-emetics are not teratogenic.

■ Corticosteroids or ondansetron may have a role to play in severe resistant cases.

Incidence

This is very common, experienced by up to 40% of women, especially in early pregnancy.

Clinical features

- Decreased frequency of defaecation
- Increased consistency of the stool, which may be fragmented and lumpy
- Increased difficulty in passing a stool
- Some women may complain of bloating, lower abdominal discomfort and increased flatus
- Constipation may well be associated with, and exacerbate, both haemorrhoids and anal fissures. Bleeding, itching, and pain on defaecation are not uncommon.

Pathogenesis

- Decreased colonic motility due to vasodilatory prostaglandins and vascular endothelial substances.
- Oral iron supplements may cause gastrointestinal upset with either constipation or diarrhoea.
- Poor fluid and food intake related to nausea and vomiting in the first trimester will exacerbate constipation.
- Pressure on the rectosigmoid colon by the gravid uterus may explain constipation in the third trimester.

Management

- Women often require reassurance that constipation is a normal feature of pregnancy.
- Advice to increase fluid intake and dietary modification with particular attention to increasing the fibre content may suffice.
- Temporary cessation of oral iron supplements may help alleviate symptoms.
- Laxatives should only be used in severe cases and if the earlier mentioned measures fail.

Laxatives

Bulk-forming drugs
Unprocessed bran, methyl cellulose, ispaghula husk or sterculia may be used in pregnancy. These should all be taken with adequate fluids to prevent intestinal obstruction.

Stimulant laxatives

Glycerol suppositories, and senna (Senokot®) tablets are safe for use in pregnancy. Danthron should be avoided.

Faecal softeners

Liquid paraffin, castor oil, and soap enemas should be avoided in pregnancy. Docusate sodium (dioctyl sodium sulphosuccinate), which acts as a stimulant as well as a softening agent, is safe for use in pregnancy.

Osmotic laxatives

Lactulose and magnesium hydrochloride are also both safe for use in pregnancy.

Reflux oesophagitis

Incidence

Oesophageal reflux is almost universal during pregnancy. Approximately 60% of women experience heartburn at some time in the third trimester.

Clinical features

- Reflux may be asymptomatic or may present with heartburn, 'water brash', nausea and vomiting, cough or wheezing, or aspiration pneumonia.
- Recurrent or forceful vomiting may cause haematemesis from a Mallory–Weiss (oesophageal mucosal) tear or abrasion.

Pathogenesis

- Decreased lower oesophageal pressure, decreased gastric peristalsis and delayed gastric emptying, all make reflux more likely.
- Later in pregnancy, the enlarging uterus exacerbates oesophageal reflux.
- Reflux of acid or alkaline gastric contents into the oesophagus causes inflammation of the oesophageal mucosa.

Management

- Antacids are safe to use in pregnancy and should be used liberally.
- Many formulations in liquid and tablet or capsule form are available. The liquid forms are more effective; they are best given to prevent symptoms before meals or at bedtime, but may be taken to relieve symptoms at any time.
- Aluminium-containing antacids tend to cause constipation and magnesium-containing antacids have a laxative effect. Both are safe for use in pregnancy.

- Reflux in late pregnancy may be relieved with postural changes, and some women find that sleeping in a sitting or semi-recumbent position will prevent symptoms at night.

- Avoiding food or fluid intake immediately before retiring at night may also help.

- Metoclopramide increases lower oesophageal pressure, speeds gastric emptying and may help relieve reflux.

- Sucralfate is also safe to use in pregnancy.

- The histamine$_2$-receptor blockers, cimetidine and ranitidine, have both been used throughout pregnancy without adverse effects, although there are theoretical reasons for preferring ranitidine, which does not interact with androgen receptors.

- Omeprazole, a proton pump inhibitor, is more effective than ranitidine or cimetidine at suppressing gastric acid secretion, and has been used in a few cases of hyperemesis. Safety data are limited but do not suggest teratogenesis. It should only be used for reflux oesophagitis when histamine$_2$-receptor blockers have failed.

Peptic ulcer disease

Incidence

- Peptic ulceration is less common in pregnant than non-pregnant women, but data may be inaccurate because of the reluctance to fully investigate symptoms of dyspepsia with endoscopy during pregnancy.

- Complications of peptic ulcer disease, such as gastrointestinal haemorrhage and perforation, are very rare in pregnancy.

Clinical features

- Epigastric pain, which may be relieved by food in the case of duodenal ulcer may be aggravated by food with a gastric ulcer.

- Heartburn and nausea make differentiation from reflux oesophagitis difficult.

- Ulcers that remain quiescent during pregnancy may cause resurgence of symptoms in the puerperium.

Pathogenesis

- Increased acid secretion and decreased mucosal resistance contribute to the aetiology.

- *Helicobacter pylori* is found in the stomach of almost 100% of patients with duodenal ulceration and is felt to have a causal role, since eradication with antibiotic therapy increases ulcer healing and decreases relapse.

■ Smoking reduces mucosal resistance.

■ The increase in prostaglandins induced by pregnancy has a protective effect on the gastric mucosa.

Diagnosis

■ A high index of suspicion is needed, but this is an uncommon diagnosis in pregnancy.

■ Although nausea, vomiting and heartburn are common in pregnancy, epigastric pain is not, and should lead the clinician to suspect a diagnosis of peptic ulcer disease. (See differential diagnosis of abdominal pain, Section B, Table 17, p. 310)

■ In experienced hands, upper gastrointestinal endoscopy can be used safely in pregnancy and should not be withheld.

■ Haematemesis, unless insubstantial, i.e. limited to one episode and not associated with a fall in haemoglobin, should be investigated with endoscopy as in the non-pregnant woman.

Management

■ Regular antacids, sucralfate and histamine$_2$ (H$_2$)-receptor blockers can all be used safely in pregnancy. Ranitidine is the most suitable H$_2$-receptor blocker.

■ *H. pylori* eradication therapy can usually be deferred until after delivery.

■ The prostaglandin analogue, misoprostol, protects the gastric mucosa, but is contraindicated during pregnancy because of the risk of inducing uterine contraction and abortion.

Inflammatory bowel disease (IBD)

This is divided into Crohn's disease and ulcerative colitis (UC).

Incidence

■ Incidence of UC is about 5–10 in 100 000 and prevalence is about 0.8 to 1 in 1000.

■ Incidence of Crohn's disease is about 5 in 100 000 and prevalence is about 0.5 in 1000.

■ UC affects more women than men, but in Crohn's disease both sexes are affected equally.

■ IBD usually presents in young adulthood.

Clinical features

Ulcerative colitis

This is always confined to the colon and causes:

- Liquid diarrhoea
- Lower abdominal pain
- Urgency of defaecation
- Passage of blood and mucus per rectum.

Crohn's disease

Crohn's disease affects the terminal ileum alone in 30%, the ileum and colon in 50%, and the colon alone in 20% of cases.

Cases with involvement of the colon may present with any of the earlier mentioned features, although bleeding is more common in UC than in Crohn's disease. Cases with ileitis present with:

- Cramping mid-abdominal pain
- Diarrhoea
- Weight loss.

Complications

Crohn's disease
- Perforation
- Stricture formation
- Peri-anal problems
- Fistulae
- Abscess formation.

Ulcerative colitis
- Colonic dilation/toxic megacolon
- Malignancy.

Extraintestinal manifestations

These include:

- Arthritis (sacroileitis, ankylosing spondylitis)
- Aphthous ulcers (Crohn's disease)
- Gallstones
- Ascending cholangitis
- Sclerosing cholangitis
- Conjunctivitis/irodocyclitis/episcleritis.

Pathogenesis

- The cause of IBD is not known.
- Infection, autoimmunity, genetic factors and environmental toxins may all be involved.
- Patchy or segmental inflammation is typical of Crohn's disease.

Diagnosis

Sigmoidoscopy or colonoscopy and mucosal biopsy confirm mucosal inflammation and allow histological examination to differentiate UC and Crohn's disease.

Pregnancy

Effect of pregnancy on IBD

- Fertility may be decreased in active Crohn's disease.
- Pregnancy has little effect on the course of IBD.
- Risk of exacerbation of UC during pregnancy is about 50% (i.e. similar to the annual risk in non-pregnant patients).
- This risk is reduced to about 30% if colitis is quiescent at the time of conception.
- Exacerbations of UC are usually mild and occur during the first two trimesters.
- Crohn's disease remains quiescent in about three-quarters of pregnant patients, and improves in about one-third of those whose disease is active at the time of conception.
- Most exacerbations of inactive Crohn's disease occur during the first trimester.
- The highest risk relates to those women with active disease at the time of conception, and those who develop IBD for the first time in pregnancy. In these instances, it usually occurs during the first or second trimesters.
- Postpartum flare of UC is no more common than in the non-pregnant patient, but may occur in Crohn's disease.

Effect of IBD on pregnancy

- In women with quiescent disease at the time of conception, the rate of miscarriage, stillbirth, fetal abnormality and livebirth are normal.
- The majority (80–90%) of women have full-term normal pregnancies.
- Active disease at the time of conception is associated with an increased miscarriage rate.

- Active disease may adversely affect pregnancy outcome, with an increased rate of prematurity.
- Women with prior surgery, including ileostomy and proctocolectomy, and pouch surgery tolerate pregnancy well. Most women with stomas and quiescent disease have full-term normal deliveries, but those with previous surgery and active disease do less well. Ileostomy dysfunction may occur in the second trimester. The most serious complication is intermittent intestinal obstruction, but peristomal cracking and bleeding may result from stretching of the abdominal wall. Successful pregnancies and vaginal deliveries have also been reported following ileoanal anastomosis.

Management

- Women should be encouraged to conceive during periods of disease remission and to avoid/postpone pregnancy if their disease is active.
- The management of acute attacks and chronic disease is not substantially affected by pregnancy.
- Deterioration of symptoms may be investigated with a full blood count, stool culture, serum albumin (allowing for the normal fall in pregnancy) and flexible sigmoidoscopy or rigid proctoscopy to assess the activity of colitis.
- Sulfasalazine (Salazopyrin®) may be safely used throughout pregnancy and breast-feeding, and is particularly used for maintaining and inducing remission in women with UC and colonic Crohn's disease. The drug is split in the colon into sulfapyridine and the active moiety 5-aminosalicylic acid. The theoretical risk of kernicterus due to displacement of bilirubin from fetal albumin has been discounted by studies. Sulfasalazine may also be used rectally.
- Sulfasalazine is a dihydrofolate reductase inhibitor that blocks the conversion of folate to its more active metabolites. The use of supplemental folic acid 5 mg/day pre-conceptually and in pregnancy is therefore important to reduce the increased risk of neural tube defects, cardiovascular defects, oral clefts, and folate deficiency.
- The closely related mesalazine (Asacol®) is also safe.
- Oral and rectal preparations of corticosteroids are also safe for use in pregnancy. For acute colonic disease, initial treatment is with topical corticosteroid enemas and oral sulfasalazine or mesalazine. Oral steroids (20–40 mg) may be required.
- Although there are extensive data regarding the safety of azathioprine in renal transplants and systemic lupus erythematosus (SLE) in pregnancy, other second-line immunosuppressive agents such as 6-mercaptopurine should be avoided (see also chapter 4, p. 63 [steroids] and chapter 8, p. 138 [azathioprine]). Those who require azathioprine to remain in remission should continue use of this drug in pregnancy.

- Metronidazole has been used extensively for other conditions in pregnancy and is safe to use.
- Rarely, surgery for obstruction, haemorrhage, perforation or toxic megacolon may be required during pregnancy, and should not be delayed because of the pregnancy.
- Caesarean section is only required for obstetric indications. In cases of severe peri-anal Crohn's disease resulting in a deformed or scarred rectum and perineum, vaginal delivery should be avoided because of perineal inelasticity. Similarly, active peri-anal Crohn's disease may prevent healing of an episiotomy.

Inflammatory bowel disease – points to remember

- Pregnancy does not usually affect the course of IBD and symptoms generally remain stable if present at conception.
- Most changes in disease activity occur early in pregnancy.
- Pregnancy outcome is not affected by quiescent IBD, but active disease at conception or during pregnancy may adversely affect the pregnancy.
- Both sulfasalazine and corticosteroids are safe to use in pregnancy and whilst breast-feeding.
- Elective caesarean section is not usually necessary, even in women with ileostomies, except for obstetric indications or in women with peri-anal Crohn's disease.

Irritable bowel syndrome (IBS)

Incidence

Irritable bowel syndrome is common, and most sufferers encountered in pregnancy will already be aware of their diagnosis. Since it is a diagnosis of exclusion, new onset of symptoms in pregnancy is more likely to be attributed to the pregnancy than to IBS.

Clinical features

- Recurrent episodes of abdominal pain, typically in the left iliac fossa, but may occur anywhere in the abdomen.
- Altered bowel habit with, most commonly constipation, but also diarrhoea.
- The history is usually long and there may be long symptom-free periods.

- The woman with IBS looks well despite frequent episodes of abdominal pain.
- There are no abnormal findings on examination.

Pathogenesis

- The cause of IBS is not known.
- Abnormal gut motility may be a contributory factor, and symptoms are usually exacerbated or brought on by stress.

Diagnosis

- IBS is a diagnosis of exclusion, and the depth of investigation depends upon the age of the patient and the length of the history.
- Most young women with a long history of intermittent abdominal pain require little in the way of invasive investigations.
- Rectal examination and sigmoidoscopy should be performed (pre-pregnancy), and although the colonic and rectal mucosa are normal, air insufflation may reproduce the pain.
- If diarrhoea is a feature, a rectal biopsy should be taken (pre-pregnancy) to exclude IBD.

Management

- Women should be reassured of the benign nature of IBS, and this in itself may help alleviate symptoms.
- Symptoms of IBS may be exacerbated by pregnancy, especially if constipation is a prominent feature.
- A high-fibre diet may help some women.
- Stool-bulking agents (see earlier) are preferred to unprocessed bran, which may worsen symptoms, in particular bloating.
- Antispasmodic agents act to relax intestinal smooth muscle and are used widely in the management of IBS in the non-pregnant woman. There is no evidence for teratogenesis with anticholinergic agents such as hyoscine (Buscopan®) and dicyclomine (Merbentyl®). Smooth muscle relaxants such as mebeverine (Colofac®) are not recommended in pregnancy.

Abdominal pain

A full differential diagnosis is given in Table 17, Section B, p. 310.

The commonest causes of abdominal pain in pregnancy are constipation and uterine contractions. The common non-obstetric surgical conditions are appendicitis, gall bladder disease and pancreatitis.

Appendicitis

Incidence

- This is the commonest non-obstetric indication for laparotomy in pregnancy.
- It usually presents in the first two trimesters with an incidence of about 1 in 3500.

Clinical features

- The symptoms and signs are similar to those in the non-pregnant woman, with abdominal pain, rebound tenderness, nausea and vomiting.
- An aggressive course with complications such as perforation, wall abscess and paralytic ileus are not uncommon, perhaps because of delay in diagnosis due to pregnancy.
- Preterm labour and perinatal mortality complicate 20% of cases with perforation.

Diagnosis

- Ultrasound has improved diagnostic accuracy and reduced the negative laparotomy rate in cases of suspected appendicitis.
- The normal appendix is not visualised in most cases.
- The inflamed appendix is characterised by an outer diameter of >6 mm, non-compressibility, lack of peristalsis or presence of a peri-appendiceal fluid collection.
- A posterolateral approach allows evaluation of the retrocaecal appendix, and transvaginal scanning that of a pelvic appendix.

Management

If the diagnosis is confirmed, a Lanz incision for appendectomy is recommended.

Gall bladder disease

Incidence

- Symptomless gallstones are detected in between 2.5% (equivalent to the incidence outside pregnancy) and 11% of pregnant women.
- Echogenic bile, or biliary sludge, may be present in over one-third of pregnant women.
- The prevalence of acute cholecystitis in pregnancy is about 0.1%.

Clinical features

- These are similar to those in the non-pregnant woman.
- Pain is present in the right upper quadrant or epigastrium, and it may radiate through to the back and tip of the scapula.
- Nausea and vomiting are common.
- Acute cholecystitis may occur at any time in pregnancy and causes more severe pain than biliary colic. There is associated tenderness and guarding in the right hypochondrium. There may be fever and shock depending on the severity of the gall bladder sepsis.
- Complications include:
  - Jaundice secondary to oedema or stones in the common bile duct
  - Pancreatitis.

Pathogenesis

- Formation of cholesterol gallstones is increased by increasing concentrations of bile cholesterol or decreasing concentrations of bile acids.
- Pregnancy and the oral contraceptive pill increase cholesterol saturation of bile and the rate of secretion of cholesterol. They also increase the ratio of cholic acid to chenoxycholic acid. The net result is increased bile lithogenicity.
- Pregnancy also impairs gall bladder contractility, leading to gall bladder stasis.
- The combination of gall bladder stasis and the secretion of lithogenic bile increases the formation of both sludge and stones during pregnancy, but both may disappear both during and after pregnancy.

Diagnosis

- Ultrasound provides a safe and accurate method of detecting gallstones.
- Acute cholecystitis is suggested if there is, in addition, a raised white blood cell count, abnormal liver function tests, pericholecystic fluid, distension and thickening of the gall bladder wall, and ultrasound transducer-induced pain over the gall bladder.
- A mildly (two-fold) raised amylase is also consistent with a diagnosis of acute cholecystitis, although greater rises suggest pancreatitis or common bile duct stones.
- The differential diagnosis of acute cholecystitis in pregnancy (see also Section B, Table 17, p. 310) includes:
  - Appendicitis (see earlier)
  - Pancreatitis (see later)
  - Peptic ulcer (see earlier)

- Pneumonia, particularly of the right lower lobe (see chapter 4, p. 67)
- Acute fatty liver of pregnancy (see chapter 11, p. 209)
- Pre-eclampsia (see chapter 1, p. 7)
- Viral hepatitis (see chapter 11, p. 200)
- Obstetric cholestasis (see chapter 11, p. 204).

Management

■ This is the same as in the non-pregnant patient.

■ Conservative management, with withdrawal of oral food and fluids, nasogastric aspiration, i.v. fluids, antibiotics and analgesia, leads to resolution of symptoms in over three-quarters of women.

■ If surgery is required, this is best done during the second trimester, when the risk of miscarriage is low and the uterus is not yet large enough to obscure or distort the surgical field.

■ Laparoscopic cholecystectomy has been safely performed in pregnancy.

■ Endoscopic removal of common bile duct stones and stent drainage in experienced hands may be performed with minimal radiation.

■ Sphincterotomy may require considerable screening time and is best deferred until after delivery.

Pancreatitis

Incidence

This rarely complicates pregnancy and the incidence is about 0.1 in 1000.

Clinical features

■ These are similar to those in the non-pregnant woman.

■ Most attacks occur in the third trimester and are mild.

■ Epigastric pain radiating through to the back with nausea and vomiting.

■ Severe pancreatitis causes pulmonary, cardiac, renal and gastrointestinal complications with shock.

Pathogenesis

■ The commonest cause of pancreatitis is gallstones and this is also the case for attacks occurring in pregnancy. The next commonest cause is alcohol.

■ Pancreatitis is not more common in pregnancy.

■ Very rarely pancreatitis in pregnancy may be precipitated by hypertriglyceridaemia, although the physiological rise in triglycerides occurring in normal pregnancy is unlikely to be sufficient to cause pancreatitis without an underlying lipid disorder.

- Primary hyperparathyroidism (see chapter 6, p. 113) is another rare cause of pancreatitis during pregnancy.

Diagnosis

- The serum amylase is invariably raised and levels >1000 U/l suggest pancreatitis or common bile duct stones.
- Pregnancy itself does not cause changes in amylase, but a raised amylase level is not specific for pancreatitis; mild elevations in amylase level occur in cholecystitis, peptic ulcer perforation and bowel obstruction.
- The absence of a diagnostic rise in serum amylase may be due to associated hyperlipidaemia that masks the rise in amylase.

Management

- There is no specific cure for pancreatitis; management should be supportive and usually involve a period of fasting with nasogastric suction if there is evidence of paralytic ileus.
- I.v. fluids and analgesia are given as required, and most cases resolve spontaneously.
- About 10% of patients may develop serious complications and an important feature of management is to identify this subgroup and ensure their rapid transfer to an intensive care unit.
- Regular monitoring of cardiovascular status, haemoglobin, white cell count, amylase, renal function, oxygen saturation, liver function, prothrombin time, glucose and calcium are essential.

Further reading

Bergin, P.S. and Harvey, P. (1992) Wernicke's encephalopathy and central pontine myelinolysis associated with hyperemesis gravidarum. *Br. Med. J.*, **305,** 517–518.

Diavcitrin, O., Park, Y.H. and Veerasuntharam, G. (1998) The safety of mesalazine in human pregnancy: a prospective cohort study. *Gastroenterology*, **114,** 23–28.

Goodwin, T.M., Montero, M. and Mestman, J.H. (1992) Transient hyperthyroidism and hyperemesis gravidarum: clinical aspects. *Am. J. Obstet. Gynecol.*, **167,** 648–652.

Hanan, I.M. (1995) Inflammatory bowel disease in pregnancy. In: Lee, R.V., Garner, P.R., Barron, W.M. and Coustan, D.R. (eds) *Current Obstetric Medicine*, Vol. 3, pp 43–58. Chicago: Mosby-Year Book.

Mazzotta, P. and Magee, L.A. (2000) A risk–benefit assessment of pharmacological and non-pharmacological treatments for nausea and vomiting of pregnancy. *Drugs*, **59**, 781–800.

Nelson-Piercy, C., Fayers, P. and de Swiet, M. (2001) Randomized, placebo-controlled trial of corticosteroids for hyperemesis gravidarum. *Br. J. Obstet. Gynaecol.*, **108**, 1–7.

Nesbitt, T.H., Kay, H.H., McCoy, M.C. and Herbert, W.N.P. (1996) Endoscopic management of biliary disease during pregnancy. *Obstet. Gynecol.*, **87**, 806–809.

Rayes, N., Neuhaus, R., David, M. et al. (1998) pregnancies following liver transplantation – how safe are they? A report of 19 cases under cyclosporine A and tacrolimus. *Clin. Transplant.*, **12**, 396–400.

CHAPTER 13
Skin disease

Physiological changes	**Co-incident conditions**
Pre-existing conditions	Acne
Eczema	Erythema nodosum
Psoriasis	Erythema multiforme
	Pityriasis rosea

Dermatoses specific to pregnancy

Polymorphic eruption

Pemphigoid gestationis

Prurigo

Pruritic folliculitis

Physiological changes

- Increased pigmentation. This begins in the first trimester and fades after delivery. Existing pigmented areas (e.g. areolae and axillae) become darker. Specific areas (e.g. linea nigrum) appear.

- Melasma is the name given to the patches of light-brown facial pigmentation developing in about 70% of women in the second half of pregnancy. The usual distribution involves the forehead, cheeks, upper lip and chin.

- Spider naevi. These occur on the face, upper trunk and arms. They can be numerous and in some cases almost confluent. Most appear in early pregnancy and regress following delivery, although 25% may persist.

- Palmar erythema. Present in up to 70% of women by the third trimester. Fades within 1 week of delivery.

- Hair fall. This is a normal feature of the postpartum period occurring in most women at between 4 and 20 weeks after delivery. It results from the increased conversion of hairs from the anagen (growing) to telogen (resting) phase, following the increased proportion of hairs in the anagen phase during pregnancy. Hair is lost diffusely, but recovery is usual within 6 months.

- Striae gravidarum. These develop in most women but are more common in obese women and those with multiple pregnancies. They appear perpendicular to skin tension lines as pink linear wrinkles. They fade and become white and atrophic, although never disappear completely.

▪ Pruritus without either rash or cholestasis can be a feature in up to 20% of normal pregnancies. Liver function tests should however be checked in any pregnant woman without a rash (other than excoriations) complaining of pruritus, especially if onset occurs in the third trimester and it involves the palms and soles (see chapter 11, p. 204 and Section B, Table 14, p. 305).

Pre-existing conditions

Eczema

▪ This often, but not invariably, improves during pregnancy. Nevertheless, since eczema and atopy are so prevalent, it remains the commonest dermatosis associated with pregnancy.

▪ Most women presenting in pregnancy have a previous history of adult or infantile asthma, eczema or atopy.

▪ Women should be reassured that if they require topical steroids to control their eczema, these are not contraindicated in pregnancy.

Psoriasis

▪ This may improve, remain unchanged or deteriorate during pregnancy. Psoriasis may present for the first time in pregnancy.

▪ Dithranol and coal tar may be safely used in pregnancy.

▪ Methotrexate is an antimetabolite and is contraindicated in pregnancy.

Rarely, a severe form of pustular psoriasis, impetigo herpetiformis, may develop. Urticated erythema, beginning in the flexures and especially the groins, is associated with sterile pustules, which may become widespread and affect mucosa. This condition is associated with severe systemic upset including fever, neutrophilia and hypocalcaemia. An increased perinatal mortality rate is also reported and these women require intensive treatment and regular fetal surveillance.

Co-incident conditions

Acne

▪ This may develop for the first time in pregnancy.

▪ Pre-existing acne may improve or worsen during pregnancy.

▪ Both tetracyclines and retinoids (vitamin A analogues, e.g. isotretinoin) are contraindicated in pregnancy. Erythromycin may be used safely.

Erythema nodosum

- This may occur in pregnancy, without any demonstrable, known underlying precipitating cause.
- Tuberculosis and sarcoidosis should be excluded with a chest X-ray. The woman should be asked about symptoms of streptococcal infection and inflammatory bowel disease, as well as any recent medication she has taken or may be taking (particularly sulphonamides).
- If no underlying cause is discovered, the prognosis is excellent.

Erythema multiforme

- This is an acute self-limiting condition predominantly affecting the peripheries.
- The symmetrical eruption consists of erythematous papules that evolve into concentric rings of varying colour with central pallor.
- Erythema multiforme may complicate pregnancy without any obvious underlying cause.
- The commoner precipitating causes should be sought (e.g. drugs and viral [particularly herpes simplex virus (HSV)] infections), before attributing the eruption to pregnancy alone.

Pityriasis rosea

- This is a self-limiting, non-recurring eruption affecting predominantly the trunk and proximal limbs.
- The lesions are reddish brown with a larger (2–6 cm) 'herald patch' preceding the development of other lesions, and may be confused with tinea because of their well-defined, scaled edge.
- Pityriasis rosea affects mainly children and young adults but may be more common in pregnancy.
- There is some evidence of a causal role for human herpes viruses.

Dermatoses specific to pregnancy

Polymorphic eruption of pregnancy (PEP) (syn. pruritic urticarial papules and plaques of pregnancy, PUPPP; toxaemic rash of pregnancy) (Fig. 13.1 A & B)

Incidence

PEP is the commonest pregnancy-specific dermatosis. The incidence is about 1 in 200–250, i.e. about 0.5%.

Clinical features

Time of onset
Third trimester, usually after 35 weeks' gestation.

Parity
More common in primiparous women and those with multiple pregnancies.

Distribution
Abdomen (with umbilical sparing), along striae, with spread to thighs, buttocks, under the breasts and upper arms.

Eruption
Pruritic, urticarial papules and plaques, rarely vesicles (but not bullae) and target lesions.

Resolution
Rapid after delivery.

Fetus

No effects on the fetus are known.

Treatment

- 1% menthol in aqueous cream.
- Most effective if kept in the fridge and applied when cold.
- 1% hydrocortisone cream or ointment. Stronger topical steroids such as Betnovate® may be required.
- Sedative antihistamine, e.g. chlorpheniramine (Piriton®) 4 mg three to four times/day or promethazine (Phenergan®) 25 mg nocte.
- Systemic steroids are only occasionally required for intractable pruritis.

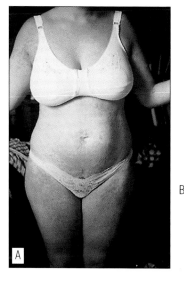

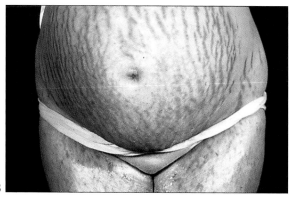

Figure 13.1A & B – Polymorphic eruption of pregnancy (PEP).

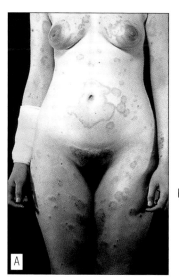

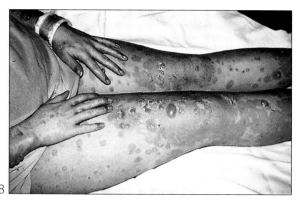

Figure 13.2A & B – Pemphigoid gestationis.

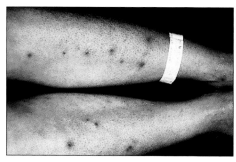

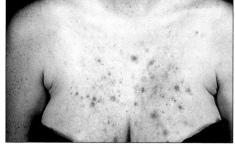

Figure 13.3 – Prurigo of pregnancy.

Figure 13.4 – Pruritic folliculitis of pregnancy.

Recurrence

Rare (mild if it occurs).

Pemphigoid gestationis (syn. herpes gestationis) (Fig. 13.2 A & B)

Incidence

This is a rare (1 in 10 000 to 1 in 60 000 pregnancies) but serious condition.

Clinical features

Time of onset
Any time (9 weeks' gestation to 1 week postpartum) but usually in the third trimester.

Parity
Primiparous or multiparous women.

Distribution
Abdomen (umbilicus affected; lesions begin in periumbilical region), spreading to limbs, palms and soles.

Eruption
Intensely pruritic; urticated erythematous papules and plaques; target lesions, annular wheals. After variable delay (usually 2 weeks) vesicles and large tense bullae form.

Resolution
If it occurs in the second trimester, there is usually an improvement at the end of pregnancy, but a flare postpartum. Urticated plaques may persist for several months after delivery.

Pathogenesis

- Autoimmune (possibly related to exposure to fetal antigens).
- Associated with bullous pemphigoid.
- Associated with other autoimmune conditions, e.g. Graves' disease, vitiligo, insulin-dependent diabetes, rheumatoid arthritis.

Diagnosis

Diagnosed by direct immunofluorescence, which shows complement (C3) deposition at the basement membrane zone. This distinguishes pemphigoid gestationis from PEP, in which immunofluorescence is negative.

Fetal considerations

- An increased risk to the fetus has been reported and studies have shown an association with low birthweight and premature delivery.
- As this is an autoimmune disease, the neonate may be affected with a similar rash, but this only occurs in 10% of cases and is mild and transient.

Treatment

- Potent topical corticosteroids (0.1% mometasone furoate, Elocon®) or very potent (0.05% clobetasol propionate, Dermovate®).
- Most require systemic steroids (e.g. prednisolone 40 mg/day and these should not be withheld in pregnancy (see chapter 4, p. 63).
- Sedative antihistamine, e.g. chlorpheniramine (Piriton®) 4 mg three to four times/day or promethazine (Phenergan®) 25 mg nocte.

Recurrence

- Usually recurs in future pregnancies (with possibly earlier onset and more severe course).
- May recur with use of combined oral contraceptive pill.

Prurigo of pregnancy (Fig. 13.3)

Incidence

1 in 300 pregnancies.

Clinical features

Time of onset
About 25–30 weeks' gestation.

Parity
Mostly multiparous women.

Distribution
Abdomen; extensor surface of limbs.

Eruption
Pruritic; groups of red/brown excoriated papules.

Resolution
Pruritus improves at delivery, but papules may sometimes persist for several months after delivery.

Pathogenesis

Associated with atopy.

Fetal considerations

No effects on the fetus are known.

Treatment

- Topical steroids (1% hydrocortisone cream or ointment).
- Antihistamines (see earlier) if required.

Recurrence

Recurrence is possible.

Pruritic folliculitis of pregnancy (Fig. 13.4)

Incidence

This is not known.

Clinical features

Time of onset
Mainly third trimester, sometimes second.

Distribution
Widespread; predominantly on the trunk, thighs and arms.

Eruption
Acneiform; pruritic; erythematous, follicular papules and pustules.

Resolution
Usually settles prior to delivery and resolves within 2 weeks after delivery.

Pathogenesis

Possibly a form of hormone-induced acne.

Fetal considerations

No effects on the fetus are known.

Treatment

- Topical 10% benzoyl peroxide
- Topical steroids (1% hydrocortisone cream or ointment)
- Antihistamines (see earlier) if required.

Further reading

Holmes, R.C. and Black, M.M. (1982) The specific dermatoses of pregnancy: a reappraisal with special emphasis on a proposed simplified classification. *Clin. Exp. Dermatol.*, **7**, 65–73.

Shornick, J.K. and Black, M.M. (1992) Fetal risks in herpes gestationis. *J. Am. Acad. Dermatol.*, **26**, 63–68.

Vaughan Jones, S.A., Hern, S., Nelson-Piercy, C., Seed, P.T. and Black, M.M. (1999) A prospective study of 200 women with dermatoses of pregnancy correlating clinical findings with hormonal and immunopathological profiles. *Br. J. Dermatol.*, **141**, 71–81.

CHAPTER 14
Haematological problems

Physiological changes	Thrombocythaemia
Anaemia	Thrombocytopenia
Haemoglobinopathies	Disseminated intravascular coagulation
Sickle-cell disease	Haemophilia and bleeding disorders
Thalassaemias	von Willebrand's disease
	Haemophilia

Haemolytic uraemic syndrome/thrombotic thrombocytopenic purpura

Physiological changes

- The plasma volume increases progressively throughout normal pregnancy.

- Most of this 50% increase occurs by 34 weeks' gestation and is positively correlated with the birthweight of the baby.

- Because the expansion in plasma volume is greater than the increase in red cell mass, there is a fall in the haemoglobin concentration, haematocrit and red cell count.

- Despite this haemodilution, there is usually no change in mean corpuscular volume (MCV) or mean corpuscular haemoglobin concentration (MCHC).

- The platelet count tends to fall progressively during normal pregnancy, although usually remains within normal limits. In a proportion of women (5–10%), the count will reach levels of $100–150 \times 10^9/l$ by term, and this may be in the absence of any pathological process. In practice therefore, a woman is not considered to be thrombocytopenic in pregnancy until the platelet count is $<100 \times 10^9/l$.

- Pregnancy causes a two- to three-fold increase in the requirement for iron, not only for haemoglobin synthesis but also for certain enzymes and for the fetus. There is a 10–20-fold increase in folate requirements.

- Changes in the coagulation system during pregnancy produce a physiological hypercoagulable state (see chapter 3, p. 40).

Anaemia

The lower limit of normal for haemoglobin concentration in the non-pregnant female is taken as 11.5–12 g/dl. In the pregnant patient, levels below 10.5 g/dl should be considered abnormal, although in certain situations such as multiple pregnancy associated with larger increases in plasma volume, the physiological dilution of haemoglobin may cause even lower concentrations of haemoglobin.

Clinical features

■ Some women begin pregnancy already anaemic and may become rapidly symptomatic.

■ Most cases present in the third trimester since this is when demands for iron reach their peak. Anaemia in pregnancy is usually diagnosed on routine testing, but may present with tiredness, lethargy, dizziness or fainting.

Pathogenesis

Iron deficiency is by far the commonest cause of anaemia and iron deficiency anaemia is the commonest haematological problem in pregnancy.

■ The increased demands for iron are met by increased intestinal absorption and by mobilising iron stores from the haemoglobin of the circulating red cells.

■ The reason why so many women not given routine iron supplementation in pregnancy become anaemic is that they enter pregnancy with depleted iron stores. Common reasons for these depleted stores include: menorrhagia, inadequate diet or previous recent pregnancies, particularly with less than a year between delivery and conception when the woman has also been breast-feeding.

■ Iron deficiency is more common in multiple pregnancy.

■ Blood loss at the time of delivery contributes to iron deficiency in the puerperium; 2–5% of women have a primary postpartum haemorrhage (blood loss >500 ml).

The next commonest cause of anaemia in pregnancy is folate deficiency.

■ The normal level of dietary folate is inadequate to prevent megaloblastic changes in the bone marrow in about 25% of pregnant women.

■ The incidence of megaloblastic anaemia is variable depending on the socio-economic status and nutrition of the population.

■ Folate deficiency is more likely if the woman is taking anticonvulsant drugs or folate antagonists such as sulfasalazine.

■ Other haematological conditions complicating pregnancy increase the risk of folate deficiency:

– Haemolytic anaemia
– Sickle-cell disease
– Thalassaemia
– Hereditary spherocytosis.

Diagnosis

Iron deficiency

■ It is generally assumed that a woman who is or becomes anaemic in pregnancy is iron deficient, but the diagnosis should be confirmed.

■ The red cell indices give a good indication of iron deficiency. The MCV, mean cell haemoglobin (MCH) and MCHC are all reduced.

■ The first index to become abnormal is the MCV, but this may be normal when stores first become depleted.

■ Serum iron and total iron binding capacity (TIBC) fall in normal pregnancy, but levels of serum iron <12 µmol/l and TIBC saturation of <15% indicate iron deficiency.

■ Serum ferritin provides an accurate assessment of iron stores; levels <12 µg/l indicate iron deficiency and levels <50 µg/l in early pregnancy are an indication for daily iron supplements.

Folate deficiency

■ This causes a macrocytic anaemia with megaloblastic change in the bone marrow.

■ The pointer is usually a raised MCV, although this may be a feature of normal pregnancy. It is also seen in azathioprine therapy and alcoholism.

■ Diagnosis is confirmed by measurement of serum and red cell folate.

Effects of iron deficiency on pregnancy

■ Iron deficiency adversely affects iron-dependent enzymes in each cell, and has profound effects on muscle and neurotransmitter activity.

■ Iron deficiency is associated with low birthweight and preterm delivery, and there is also an association with increased blood loss at delivery.

Management

■ The rationale for routine supplementation with oral iron is that the increased iron demand during pregnancy cannot be met by increased absorption alone, and that a high proportion of women in their reproductive years lack storage iron.

- Iron supplements prevent iron deficiency anaemia. Many argue that the best approach to iron deficiency in pregnancy is prevention.

- The World Health Organisation in conjunction with the International Nutritional Anemia Consultative Group and the United Nations Children's Fund have issued guidelines recommending routine supplements (60 mg/day iron and 400 μg/day folic acid) to all pregnant women for at least 6 months. The guidelines also state that these supplements should be recommended to women until 3 months postpartum in areas with a high prevalence of anaemia (>40%).

- The standard oral preparations (Pregaday®: 100 mg iron, 350 μg folate; Fefol®) are combined with folic acid and are suitable for both prevention and treatment of iron deficiency in pregnancy.

- Iron absorption from the small intestine is enhanced by ascorbic acid, meat and alcohol. Inhibitors to absorption include phytic acid and tannins present in tea, coffee and chocolate.

- The incidence of gastrointestinal side effects (30%) is directly related to the dose of iron taken. A dose of 60 mg/day (or even weekly) of iron may be sufficient for prophylaxis. Therefore women who have troublesome side effects may be advised to take alternate day or weekly supplements rather than to discontinue them.

- For those women who are unable to tolerate oral preparations, parenteral therapy (i.m., or more recently i.v.) is an option, but this does not provide more rapid correction of iron deficiency.

- Iron deficiency diagnosed late in pregnancy may necessitate blood transfusion as the maximum rise in haemoglobin achievable with either oral or parenteral iron is 0.8 g/dl/week.

- Similar arguments apply to routine folate supplementation in pregnancy, since a normal diet is not sufficient enough to meet the increased requirement for folate in pregnancy.

- All women planning a pregnancy are now advised to take 0.4 mg/day folate periconceptually as a prophylactic agent against neural tube defects and other fetal abnormalities.

- In addition, women who themselves have spina bifida, who have had a previous fetus with a neural tube defect or who are taking anticonvulsants or sulfasalazine are advised to take 5 mg/day folate periconceptually.

- The 5 mg/day dose is also appropriate for those with other haematological problems (see earlier), those with established folate deficiency, and women with diabetes.

- Vitamin B_{12} injections may be safely continued in pregnancy.

Anaemia – points to remember

- The plasma volume increases by 50% in pregnancy and there is a fall in haemoglobin concentration.
- Pregnancy causes a two- to three-fold increase in the requirement for iron, and a 10–20-fold increase in folic acid requirements.
- Many women develop iron deficiency anaemia because they enter pregnancy with depleted iron stores.
- A woman may be iron deficient despite having a normal haemoglobin level and MCV.
- The best approach to iron and folate deficiency in pregnancy is prevention with oral iron and folate supplements, at least in those at high risk of becoming anaemic.
- All women planning a pregnancy should be advised to take 0.4 mg/day folate periconceptually as a prophylactic agent against neural tube defects and other fetal abnormalities.
- The maximum rise in haemoglobin achievable with either oral or parenteral iron is 0.8 g/dl/week.

Haemoglobinopathies

Sickle-cell disease

Incidence

This varies enormously around the UK, but most cases are concentrated in urban areas. Sickle-cell trait (HbAS) is much more common, but other than implications for genetic counselling (see later) does not affect pregnancy in the same way as sickle-cell disease.

Clinical features

- Anaemia (not marked in women with HbSC disease)
- Painful crises
- Infections. The increased risk of infections is partly due to loss of splenic function
- Acute chest syndrome. This is characterised by fever, tachypnoea, pleuritic chest pain, leukocytosis and pulmonary infiltrates. It may be caused by pulmonary infection or infarction from intravascular sickling or thrombosis
- Splenic sequestration
- Retinopathy

254

- Leg ulcers
- Aseptic necrosis of bone
- Renal papillary necrosis
- Stroke.

Pathogenesis

- Sickle-cell haemoglobin (HbS) is a variant of the β-chain of haemoglobin. Sickling of the red cells occurs particularly in response to hypoxia, cold, acidosis and dehydration.
- Intravascular sickling leads to vaso-occlusive symptoms and tissue infarction with severe pain.
- A number of sickling conditions exist:
  - Homozygous sickle-cell disease (HbSS)
  - Sickle cell/HbC (HbSC)
  - Sickle-cell thalassaemia.
- Those with HbSS have chronic haemolytic anaemia, but are generally healthy except during periods of crisis, which are often precipitated by infection. A generalised vasculopathy or massive sickling leads to premature death at a mean age below 50 years.
- Those with HbSC are not usually very anaemic, but are still at risk of sickling. They also have a reduced life expectancy (68 years). They are particularly at risk in pregnancy because doctors and midwives may be unaware of the risk of sickling and have a false sense of security because of the absence of severe anaemia.

Diagnosis

Most women enter pregnancy with the diagnosis established, but if there is doubt, the diagnosis may be made by haemoglobin electrophoresis.

Effect of pregnancy on sickle-cell disease

- Complications of sickle-cell disease are more common in pregnancy.
- Crises complicate about 35% of pregnancies in women with sickle-cell disease.

Effect of sickle-cell disease on pregnancy

- Perinatal mortality is increased four- to six-fold.
- There is an increased incidence of miscarriage, intrauterine growth restriction (IUGR), premature labour, pre-eclampsia (which may have an early onset and an accelerated course), fetal distress and caesarean section.

- Sickling infarcts in the placenta may be responsible for some of these factors, although maternal anaemia and increased blood viscosity could also contribute to the high incidence of IUGR.
- There is an increased risk of pulmonary thrombosis, thromboembolism and bone marrow embolism.
- Maternal morbidity and mortality are increased and the latter has been estimated to be 2.5%.
- There is also an increased risk of infection, particularly urinary tract infection, pneumonia and puerperal sepsis.

Management

- Antenatal care should take place in combined clinics with haematologists and obstetricians experienced in the management of these disorders.
- Folic acid (5 mg/day) and penicillin prophylaxis should be given to all women.
- Electrophoresis will determine the level of HbF (the higher the level the better the outcome) and the percentage of HbS.
- If pre-pregnancy genetic counselling and screening of the partner has not already been undertaken, this should be advised in order to determine the risk of the baby having HbSS (50% if the partner is sickle-cell trait).
- Haemoglobin and mid-stream urine should be checked at each visit.
- Regular ultrasound assessment of fetal growth should be undertaken, with 2–4 weekly growth parameters and umbilical artery Doppler blood-flow assessment from 24 weeks' gestation.
- Crises should be managed aggressively as in the non-pregnant patient. This involves admission, adequate pain relief with i.v. or s.c. infusions of morphine, adequate rehydration and early use of antibiotics if infection is suspected.
- The patient should be kept warm and well oxygenated. Arterial blood gases or pulse oximetry are mandatory, especially in the context of high doses of opiates.
- In the acute chest syndrome, it may be necessary to treat the patient with both heparin and antibiotics.
- Blood transfusion may be required for severe anaemia, splenic sequestration or in acute chest syndrome. Exchange transfusion may be necessary if the patient is volume replete.
- The role of routine exchange transfusion in pregnancy is controversial. Proponents claim a decrease in the number of crises, although there is little evidence for improved fetal outcome. The risks include:
  - Delayed and immediate transfusion reactions
  - Precipitation of a crisis (particularly if the haematocrit level is raised above 0.35 l/l)

- Infection
- Red cell antibodies (because the donor blood is often from people of a different ethnic origin from the patient)
- Iron overload.

■ Caesarean section should only be performed for obstetric indications and general anaesthesia should be avoided if possible, especially if the patient has not been transfused.

Pre-pregnancy counselling

Ideally, partners of those with sickle-cell disease or trait should be screened prior to pregnancy in order to give couples an accurate estimate of the risk of having an affected child.

In practice, much of the screening of partners is performed during pregnancy, by which time it may be too late for prenatal screening of the fetus by chorionic villus sampling. Later screening with amniocentesis or fetal blood sampling may be the only options for prenatal diagnosis.

Sickle-cell disease – points to remember

■ Antenatal care should involve haematologists and obstetricians with expertise in the management of such pregnancies.

■ Complications of sickle-cell disease, particularly crises, are more common in pregnancy.

■ Perinatal and maternal morbidity and mortality rates are increased.

■ The risks for the baby include miscarriage, IUGR and prematurity.

■ The risks for the mother include thrombosis, severe pre-eclampsia, infection, and transfusion reactions.

■ Folic acid (5 mg/day) should be given to all women.

■ Infection, hypoxia, acidosis and dehydration should be prevented and treated aggressively.

■ Prophylactic exchange transfusion may decrease the risk of crises, but carries its own risks.

Thalassaemias

Incidence

■ These inherited disorders of globin synthesis are divided into two main groups, the α-thalassaemias where one to four of the α-genes are deleted, and the β-thalassaemias where one or two of the β-globin genes are defective.

- α-thalassaemia is common in South-East Asians, and β-thalassaemia is common in Cypriots and Asians.
- The overall carrier rate in the UK for β-thalassaemia is about 1 in 10 000 people, but again there are marked local variations depending on the ethnic mix of the population.

Clinical features

- α-thalassaemia trait is either α^+ (three normal α-genes) or α^0 (two normal α-genes). Such individuals are usually asymptomatic, but it is important to identify particularly those with α^0, since they may become anaemic.
- α-thalassaemia major results if both parents have α^0 and there are no functional α-genes. This condition is incompatible with life and the fetus becomes severely hydropic.
- Women with β-thalassaemia trait are asymptomatic, but as in α-thalassaemia may become anaemic during pregnancy.
- Those with β-thalassaemia major have inherited a defective β-globin gene from each parent. Without regular transfusions, this condition is usually fatal within a few years, but children can now survive into the second or third decade. The clinical features are iron overload (due to repeated transfusions) resulting in hepatic, endocrine and cardiac dysfunction, and bone deformities due to expansion of bone marrow, especially in those who are not transfused regularly. Bone marrow transplantation is now another option for these patients. Pregnancy is very rare in women with β-thalassaemia major, but is more likely in those with less iron overload who have survived without regular transfusion.

Diagnosis

- The diagnosis of α- or β-thalassaemia trait may be suspected by finding a low MCV, a low MCH and a normal MCHC (as distinct from iron deficiency when all the indices are reduced).
- The diagnosis is confirmed by globin chain synthesis studies, DNA analysis or, in the case of β-thalassaemia, raised concentrations of HbA_2 and HbF (excess α-chains combined with δ- or γ-chains because of the lack of β-chains).

Management

- Women with α- or β-thalassaemia trait need iron and folate oral supplements throughout pregnancy, but should not be given parenteral iron.
- If both parents have α^0- or β-thalassaemia trait, the woman should be referred for prenatal diagnosis since there is a risk that the fetus may have α- or β-thalassaemia major.

- If anaemia does not respond to oral iron and folate, i.m. folate may be given, but transfusion may be required prior to delivery.

Thrombocythaemia

Incidence

Essential thrombocythaemia, causing an isolated thrombocytosis, is a myeloproliferative disorder and is rare in women of child-bearing age.

Clinical features

The high platelet count may be associated with both haemorrhagic and thromboembolic manifestations.

Diagnosis

- The diagnosis is usually made pre-pregnancy.
- A high platelet count may be discovered during pregnancy in women who have undergone traumatic or therapeutic splenectomy, especially if they are also anaemic.
- Other typical features will accompany the thrombocytosis on blood film examination.
- Differential diagnosis includes infection and inflammation and postsurgical acute phase response.

Effects of thrombocythaemia on pregnancy

Women with essential thrombocytosis have an increased risk of adverse pregnancy outcome, possibly related to placental thrombosis, including IUGR.

Management

- The platelet count may fall and even normalise spontaneously in pregnancy.
- If the count is $>600 \times 10^9/l$, treatment with low-dose aspirin (75 mg/day) is warranted. This inhibits platelet aggregation and thrombosis.
- Outside pregnancy cytotoxic agents are used for myelosuppression, but these should be avoided in pregnancy.
- Interferon-α is also used for myelosuppression in this condition, and this may be safely continued or instituted in pregnancy.

Thrombocytopenia

Causes of thrombocytopenia in pregnancy

- Spurious result (reduced platelets on automated Coulter counter due to platelet clumping or misreading of large immature platelets as red cells)
- Gestational thrombocytopenia
- Immune thrombocytopenic purpura (ITP)
- Pre-eclampsia and Haemolysis, Elevated Liver enzymes and Low Platelets (HELLP) syndrome (see chapter 1, p. 8)
- Disseminated intravascular coagulation (DIC); see later
- Haemolytic uraemic syndrome (HUS)/thrombotic thrombocytopenic purpura (TTP); see later
- Human immunodeficiency virus (HIV), drugs and infections (see chapter 15, p. 269)
- Systemic lupus erythematosus (SLE) and antiphospholipid syndrome (APS) (see chapter 8, pp 140 and 146)
- Bone marrow suppression.

ITP and gestational thrombocytopenia are considered in this section.

Incidence

- 5–10% of pregnant women may have thrombocytopenia at term, but at least 75% of these women have 'pregnancy-associated' or 'gestational' thrombocytopenia.
- Chronic ITP usually affects young women (female to male ratio = 3:1) and is quite commonly encountered in pregnancy, with an estimated incidence of 1–2 in 10 000 pregnancies.
- Alloimmune thrombocytopenia is a fetal disorder caused by feto-maternal incompatibility for platelet antigens (similar to Rhesus haemolytic disease of the newborn). There are no maternal symptoms and the mother is not thrombocytopenic. The condition develops *in utero*, affects all children including the first born, but is usually (except in the case of subsequent siblings) diagnosed after birth. The incidence is about 1 in 2000 and it causes about 10% of all cases of neonatal thrombocytopenia.

Clinical features

- Gestational thrombocytopenia is a benign condition and even if the platelet count falls to $<100 \times 10^9/l$, there are no adverse consequences for mother or baby.
- Haemorrhage in ITP is unlikely with platelet counts $>50 \times 10^9/l$, and spontaneous haemorrhage without surgery is unlikely with counts $>20 \times 10^9/l$.

Patients may present with skin bruising or gum bleeding but severe haemorrhage is rare.

■ Thrombocytopenia documented in the first half of pregnancy is less likely to be due to the pregnancy itself and should alert the clinician to a possible diagnosis of ITP.

■ In ITP, there is isolated thrombocytopenia without any associated haematological abnormality. There is no splenomegaly or lymphadenopathy.

Pathogenesis

Gestational thrombocytopenia

The platelet count tends to fall progressively during normal pregnancy and in 5–10% of women, the count will reach thrombocytopenic levels $(50–150 \times 10^9/l)$ by term.

ITP

Autoantibodies against platelet surface antigens cause peripheral platelet destruction by the reticuloendothelial system, particularly the spleen.

Diagnosis

■ In specialist laboratories, differentiation between ITP and 'essential thrombocytopenia of pregnancy' is possible with antiplatelet antibody determination, but the assay is not readily available.

■ The diagnosis of ITP is one of exclusion, and should only be made once other causes of thrombocytopenia (see earlier), such as infection and pre-eclampsia, have been excluded.

■ In ITP, the bone marrow is normal or megakaryocytic, but a bone marrow examination is not necessary in pregnancy in cases of isolated thrombocytopenia unless it is severe (platelet count $<30 \times 10^9/l$).

Effect of pregnancy on ITP

Pregnancy does not affect the course of ITP, but anxieties arise around the time of delivery because of possible bleeding associated with vaginal and abdominal delivery and regional anaesthesia and analgesia.

Effect of ITP on pregnancy

■ Capillary bleeding and purpura are unlikely with a platelet count of $>50 \times 10^9/l$, and spontaneous mucous membrane bleeding is not a risk with platelet counts $>20 \times 10^9/l$.

- Antiplatelet IgG can cross the placenta and cause fetal thrombocytopenia. Accurate prediction of the fetal platelet count from the maternal platelet count, antibody level or splenectomy status is not possible, so it is difficult to predict which fetuses will be affected.

- The level of risk to the fetus, which has been overestimated in older studies, is small, unlike the fetal risk in alloimmune thrombocytopenia.

- The risk of fetal platelet counts $<50 \times 10^9/l$ is about 5–10%, although it may be higher in women known to have ITP before pregnancy and in those with symptomatic ITP in the index pregnancy.

- The incidence of antenatal or neonatal intracranial haemorrhage in women with ITP may reach 2%, but in the absence of maternal symptoms or a history of ITP prior to the index pregnancy, the fetal risk is even lower.

- One of the best predictors of severe neonatal thrombocytopenia is a previously affected child, and the incidence of serious haemorrhage in the fetus and neonate is low.

Management

Gestational thrombocytopenia

This benign condition requires no intervention.

ITP

Maternal considerations
- Exclude associated conditions such as SLE or APS.
- The platelet count should be monitored fortnightly to monthly.
- Treatment is required in pregnancy for symptomatic thrombocytopenia (usually with counts $<20 \times 10^9/l$).
- Counts $<50 \times 10^9/l$, even in the absence of bleeding, probably warrant prophylactic treatment prior to delivery.
- Caesarean section is only required for obstetric indications and epidural and spinal anaesthesia is safe with stable counts $>80 \times 10^9/l$. The bleeding time does not predict haemorrhage and is not indicated.
- Corticosteroids are the first-line therapy, and high doses (60–80 mg/day, 1 mg/kg/day) of prednisolone are usually given until a response is obtained. Following this, the dose may be weaned to the lowest that will maintain a satisfactory ($>50 \times 10^9/l$) maternal platelet count.
- I.v. gamma-globulin may be used in resistant cases, in women likely to require prolonged therapy, in women requiring a high maintenance dose of prednisolone or in those who are intolerant of prednisolone.
- I.v. immunoglobulin is thought to work by delaying clearance of IgG-coated

platelets from the maternal circulation. The response is more rapid (24–48 hours) than with steroids, and lasts for 2–3 weeks, but immunoglobulin is expensive and seldom produces long-term remission. It is useful in pregnancy if a rapid response is required. There is also concern about the transmission of unknown viruses and hepatitis C has been transmitted with i.v. immunoglobulin. Therefore only preparations that have undergone a validated viral inactivation procedure should be used.

■ Possible dose regimes would be 0.4 g/kg/day for 5 days or 1 g/kg over 8 hours repeated 2 days later if there is an inadequate response.

■ Splenectomy should be avoided in pregnancy if possible, but may be necessary in extreme cases. Women with ITP who have previously been treated with splenectomy, should continue penicillin prophylaxis throughout pregnancy.

■ Other options for women who fail to respond to oral prednisolone and immunoglobulin include i.v. methylprednisolone or azathioprine. Although not recommended, danazol and vincristine have been successfully used for severe resistant cases in pregnancy.

■ Platelet transfusions are given as a last resort for bleeding or prior to surgery; they will increase antibody titres.

Fetal considerations

■ The transfer of IgG increases at the end of pregnancy and the baby is not at risk of bleeding before labour and delivery, so there is no place for serial fetal blood samples earlier in gestation.

■ Caesarean section is only indicated for obstetric reasons. The risk of fetal blood sampling via cordocentesis (cord spasm, haemorrhage from the cord puncture site) is similar (or even higher in thrombocytopenic fetuses) to the risk of intracerebral haemorrhage (ICH). There is no conclusive evidence that caesarean section reduces the incidence of ICH, or that it is less traumatic for the fetus than vaginal delivery.

Immune thrombocytopenia – points to remember

■ The diagnosis of ITP is one of exclusion and should only be made once other causes of thrombocytopenia have been excluded.

■ Bleeding is unlikely if the platelet count is $>50 \times 10^9/l$.

■ The risk of serious thrombocytopenia and haemorrhage in the neonate from transplacental passage of antiplatelet IgG is low.

■ Caesarean section is only required for obstetric indications and epidural and spinal anaesthesia is safe with stable counts $>80 \times 10^9/l$.

■ Treatment, if required, should be with corticosteroids or i.v. immunoglobulin.

- Cord platelet count is determined immediately after delivery, but the neonatal platelet count only reaches a nadir after 2–5 days in affected infants, when splenic circulation is established; therefore monitoring is necessary over this time. I.v. gammaglobulin is the recommended treatment for neonates with bleeding or severe thrombocytopenia; this may be given prophylactically if the platelet count of the cord blood is low ($<20 \times 10^9/l$).

Disseminated intravascular coagulation (DIC)

Obstetric causes of DIC

- Haemorrhage (particularly abruption)
- Pre-eclampsia, HELLP syndrome
- Amniotic fluid embolism
- Massive infection, particularly intrauterine infection
- Retention of a dead fetus.

Clinical features

DIC may be asymptomatic or associated with massive haemorrhage depending on the degree.

Pathogenesis

- Procoagulant substances, such as thromboplastin, phospholipid, and those resulting from endothelial injury are released into the circulation and cause stimulation of coagulation activity with increased production and breakdown of coagulation factors.
- Consumption of clotting factors and platelets leads to bleeding.
- Fibrinolysis is stimulated and fibrinogen degradation products (FDPs) interfere with the production of firm fibrin clots, so exacerbating bleeding.

Diagnosis

The *in vitro* diagnosis of DIC is made by finding:

- ↑ FDPs (these may be elevated postdelivery)
- ↑ Soluble fibrin complexes
- ↓ Fibrinogen (fibrinogen concentration is normally elevated in mid- and late pregnancy so a level <2 g/l is highly significant)
- ↓ Platelets
- Prolongation of clotting times (thrombin time, activated partial thromboplastin time, prothrombin time).

Management

Management of DIC can be considered as the treatment of the underlying cause and treatment of haemorrhage and coagulopathy.

- This usually necessitates delivery of the fetus and emptying of the uterus.
- Pregnancy may be prolonged in cases of mild DIC associated with pre-eclampsia at early gestational ages, but such conservative management necessitates very careful monitoring.
- The obstetric patient with massive bleeding should be managed according to pre-defined and agreed protocols in close collaboration with haematology and anaesthetic staff. Guidelines for the management of massive obstetric haemorrhage can be found in the Report on Confidential Enquiries into Maternal Deaths 1988–1990 (see Further reading, Department of Health, 1994). Adequate monitoring with a central venous pressure line and urinary catheter is essential.

The coagulopathy is treated with the following:

- Fresh frozen plasma (FFP), which contains all the coagulation factors
- Red cells (only needed to replace losses)
- Platelet concentrates (may be given to a bleeding patient if the platelet count is $<80 \times 10^9/l$)
- Cryoprecipitate (contains more fibrinogen than FFP but lacks antithrombin. Its use may be considered if there is haemorrhage and the fibrinogen concentration is <1 g/l).

The coagulation disturbance usually resolves within 24–48 hours after delivery, although thrombocytopenia may persist for up to a week postpartum.

Haemophilia and bleeding disorders

von Willebrand's disease

- This is the most common inherited bleeding disorder (incidence about 1%).
- von Willebrand factor (vWf) is a large multivalent adhesive protein that has important roles in platelet function and stability of factor VIII.
- There are several different types of von Willebrand's disease, involving complete or partial deficiency of, or defective vWf.
- Inheritance is different for the different types of the disease.
- Those with von Willebrand's disease may present with menorrhagia, epistaxis, bleeding after dental extraction or postoperative bleeding.
- vWf antigen is usually low, the bleeding time may be prolonged and factor VIII levels are low in some types.
- Pregnancy, labour and the puerperium are associated with significant bleeding problems but these are largely preventable.

- Pregnancy may lead to normalisation of vWf antigen and factor VIII levels.
- In some cases desmopressin (DDAVP) to increase vWf levels may be indicated, for example prior to surgical procedures.
- Rarely, vWf concentrate may be used to control severe bleeding.

Haemophilia

- Haemophilia A (factor VIII deficiency) and haemophilia B (factor IX deficiency) are rare X-linked recessive disorders.
- Some female carriers may be symptomatic, in which case DDAVP or factor VIII concentrates may be indicated for haemophilia A or tranexamic acid or factor IX concentrate for haemophilia B. Close liaison with the haemophilia centre is essential.

Haemolytic uraemic syndrome (HUS)/thrombotic thrombocytopenic purpura (TTP)

- Thrombotic thrombocytopenic purpura and haemolytic uraemic syndrome are a continuum. Both are manifestations of a similar mechanism of microvascular platelet aggregation.
- The common features are thrombocytopenia, assumed to be a consequence of platelet consumption at sites of endothelial injury, and microangiopathic haemolytic anaemia.
- If this is systemic and extensive – and especially if there is central nervous system involvement – the disorder is TTP.
- If platelet aggregation is relatively less extensive, with predominantly renal involvement, the disorder is HUS.
- Both TTP and HUS are rare during pregnancy and the puerperium.
- 'Idiopathic renal failure of pregnancy' was probably a manifestation of HUS.

Clinical features

- It is seen most commonly in the immediate postnatal period.
- The classic 'pentad of TTP' is:
  - Microangiopathic haemolytic anaemia
  - Thrombocytopenia
  - Fever
  - Neurological manifestations
  - Renal impairment.
- The clinical features of TTP/HUS may be confused with pre-eclampsia and particularly HELLP syndrome. However, hypertension is not common in TTP/HUS.

- Features include headache, irritability, drowsiness, seizures, coma and fever.
- The condition is usually severe and associated with increased maternal morbidity and mortality.

Pathogenesis

- These conditions involve a thrombotic microangiopathy, where aggregates of platelets reversibly obstruct the arterioles and capillaries.
- The association with pregnancy may perhaps be due to the formation of endothelial cell autoantibodies associated with immune dysregulation during pregnancy.
- There is diffuse vascular endothelial insult. Endothelial cells secrete unusually large forms of vWF. These large multimers agglutinate platelets.
- TTP is associated with deficiency of a specific vWF-cleaving protease (metalloprotease).
- In non-familial TTP there is an inhibitor of vWf-cleaving protease.
- In familial TTP there is a constitutional deficiency of vWf-cleaving protease.
- In HUS there is no deficiency.
- It is likely that TTP/HUS are both on a continuum with pre-eclampsia and HELLP syndrome as all conditions are characterised by widespread endothelial cell injury. In some cases HELLP syndrome may 'evolve' into HUS.

Diagnosis

- Microangiopathic haemolytic anaemia with red cell fragments (schistocytes) on the blood film.
- Thrombocytopenia, which may be severe.
- Depending on the degree of haemolysis, there is anaemia, increased reticulocytes and increased unconjugated bilirubin and lactate dehydrogenase.
- In HUS, there is impaired renal function, which may be severe.
- Clotting times and fibrinogen concentrations are normal. A consumptive coagulopathy (DIC) is rare in HUS/TTP, unless there is associated septicaemia (see also p. 196 for differential diagnosis of thrombocytopenia and acute renal failure, and Section B, Table 13, p. 303 for differential diagnosis of abnormal renal function.)

Effect of TTP on pregnancy

The fetus is not affected by TTP and prognosis is related to the gestational age at delivery.

Management

■ There is no evidence that delivery affects the course of TTP and HUS, which is why differentiation from DIC and pre-eclampsia is important (see chapter 11, p. 213).

■ Aggressive treatment with FFP and plasmapheresis may limit vascular injury and improve prognosis.

■ Corticosteroids may be of benefit.

■ Antiplatelet therapy is also used, but is more controversial.

■ Supportive therapy for renal impairment, which may necessitate dialysis in addition to plasmapheresis.

■ Supportive therapy for cerebral involvement, which may include investigation to exclude other causes of seizures (see chapter 9, p. 157 and Section B, Table 8, p. 296).

■ Platelet transfusions are contraindicated.

Further reading

Burrows, R.F. and Kelton, J.G. (1993) Fetal thrombocytopenia and its relation to maternal thrombocytopenia. *N. Engl. J. Med.*, **329**, 1463–1466.

Department of Health (1994) Revised guidelines for the management of massive obstetric haemorrhage. Annexe to Ch. 3, pp 43–44. Report on Confidential Enquiries into Maternal Deaths in the UK 1988–1990. London: HMSO.

Economides, D.L. and Kadir, R.A. (1999) Inherited bleeding disorders in obstetrics and gynaecology. *Br. J. Obstet. Gynaecol.*, **106**, 5–13.

Furlan, M., Robles, R., Galbusera, M. et al. (1998) Von Willebrand factor-cleaving protease in thrombotic thrombocytopenic purpura and the haemolytic-uraemic syndrome. *N. Engl. J. Med.*, **339**, 1578–1584.

Howard, R.J. (1996) Management of sickling conditions in pregnancy. *Br. J. Hosp. Med.*, **56**, 7–10.

Letsky, E.A. and Greaves, M. on behalf of the Maternal and Neonatal Haemostasis and Thrombosis Task Force of the British Society for Haematology (1996). Guidelines on the Investigation and Management of Thrombocytopenia in Pregnancy and Neonatal Alloimmune Thrombocytopenia. *Br. J. Haematol.*, **95**, 21–26.

Nield, G.H. (1994) Haemolytic-uraemic syndrome in practice. *Lancet*, **343**, 398–401.

Pillai, M. (1993) Platelets and pregnancy. *Br. J. Obstet. Gynaecol.*, **100**, 201–204.

Stoltzfus, R.J. and Dreyfuss, M.I. (1998) Guidelines for the use of iron supplements to prevent and treat iron deficiency anemia. International Nutritional Anemia Consultative Group, World Health Organisation, United Nations Children's Fund. Washington: ILSI Press.

CHAPTER 15

Human immunodeficiency virus and other infectious diseases

HIV	Listeriosis
Other viral infections	Malaria

Human immunodeficiency virus (HIV)

Incidence

- The incidence of HIV infection is increasing worldwide; 43% of infected adults are women, of which 80% are of child-bearing age.
- In 1998 a total of over 33 million people worldwide were infected.
- Two-thirds of those infected live in sub-Saharan Africa; about one-quarter are children.
- Prevalence rates in pregnancy vary enormously geographically. In the UK, anonymous testing in the early 1990s showed rates of 0.16% in inner London and 0.25% in Edinburgh. More recent surveys have shown rates of 0.5% in inner London. Much higher rates exist in Zaire (5%), Kenya (13%) and Uganda (30%).
- Perinatal transmission rates average from 25–30% but are also very variable (see later).
- In the UK, about 300 HIV-infected women give birth each year.

Clinical features

- Because of advances in drug therapy, HIV infection is now regarded in the developed world as a carrier state or chronic infection.

- Acute, primary infection, or seroconversion may be asymptomatic or accompanied by fever, fatigue, lymphadenopathy or rash. This usually occurs 2 weeks to 3 months after exposure to the virus.
- A clinically latent phase then follows, lasting up to and beyond 10 years.
- Symptomatic disease includes persistent generalised lymphadenopathy, weight loss, fever, diarrhoea, neurological disease including encephalopathy and neuropathy, and a range of opportunistic infections and secondary cancers including:
  - *Pneumocystis* pneumonia
  - Cerebral toxoplasmosis
  - Cytomegalovirus (CMV) retinitis
  - *Mycobacterium tuberculosis* and *Mycobacterium avium-intracellulare*
  - Kaposi's sarcoma
  - non-Hodgkin's lymphoma
  - Candidiasis
  - *Cryptococcus.*
- In countries that are able to provide highly active antiretroviral treatments (HAARTs), HIV-associated morbidity and mortality have declined significantly, although clinical progression continues to occur.

Pathogenesis

In the UK, 28% of HIV infection is acquired by heterosexual transmission and 60% by male homosexual intercourse.

The virus is transmitted by three principal routes:

- *Sexual:* unprotected anal or vaginal intercourse, especially in the presence of genital ulceration
- *Parenteral* (blood-borne): sharing of contaminated needles, unscreened blood products
- *Perinatal:* vertical transmission (see later) either antepartum, intrapartum, or postpartum (breast milk).

Early HIV infection is characterised by a high viral load. The main target of HIV is the CD4 lymphocyte population and lymphocytes are gradually lost during the latent phase. Loss of CD4 lymphocytes reduces both cell-mediated immunity and humoral immunity, leading to the development of infections and allowing more rapid replication of HIV.

Diagnosis

- The HIV antibody test detects an antibody to part of the viral membrane or envelope.

- The test usually becomes positive within 3 weeks to 3 months after exposure, as levels of p24 antigen are falling.
- Viral DNA and RNA detection are possible with the polymerase chain reaction (PCR).
- The hallmark of HIV infection is the progressive decline in CD4 lymphocyte count, which falls by about 60 cells/mm^3/year.
- The CD4 count indicates the current degree of immunosuppression.
- The viral load (HIV-RNA) is the main predictor of the speed of disease progression. Other correlates of disease progression are low levels of p24 antibodies and recurrence of p24 antigen.
- Transplacental transfer of maternal HIV antibody may persist for up to 18 months, making true HIV status of the infant difficult to determine without the use of PCR.
- The standard for diagnosis of HIV infection in exposed infants is viral assays (HIV-DNA PCR [preferred], HIV-RNA PCR or viral culture) obtained within 48 hours of birth, 1–2 months, and 3–6 months of age.

Screening

- Although up to 1 in 200 pregnant women in inner London may be HIV positive, only 20% are aware of their status.
- There are interventions of proven efficacy available during pregnancy to decrease the risk of vertical transmission (see later).
- It is important that at-risk infants are identified to allow for careful monitoring, prophylaxis and early treatment of infection.
- Knowledge of HIV status may influence women's plans regarding pregnancy.
- Early treatment of HIV-positive women improves long-term outcome.
- Knowledge of HIV status allows for protection of sexual partners.
- High-risk groups of women include:
  - I.v. drug users
  - Sex workers
  - Haemophiliacs
  - Workmen from sub-Saharan Africa
  - Partners of individuals in any of the above groups or of homosexual/bisexual males.
- Policies of selective screening of high-risk women have failed.
- National policy is to offer and recommend HIV screening in early pregnancy to all women, and to make such testing an integral and accepted part of antenatal care. Pre- and post-test counselling are important parts of such a screening policy. The aim is to increase the uptake of HIV testing to 90%.

Pregnancy

Effect of pregnancy on HIV disease

- Pregnancy probably does not have a major adverse effect on HIV progression in asymptomatic women.
- Women with advanced disease are at high risk of deterioration in the short term, but this is probably not accelerated by pregnancy.
- Opportunistic infection in pregnancy may be less aggressively investigated or treated due to concerns regarding the fetus, and this may indirectly worsen prognosis for the HIV-infected mother.
- Opportunistic infection may be less aggressively investigated or treated as many of the symptoms may mimic symptoms of pregnancy (e.g. breathlessness). This is more likely if HIV status is unknown and HIV positivity unsuspected.
- Normal pregnancy is associated with a depression of cell-mediated immunity and a fall in the CD4 lymphocyte count, although the percentage of CD4 cells is unchanged. Similar changes occur in HIV-infected pregnant women.
- There is no evidence to suggest that pregnancy increases the risk of progression to acquired immune deficiency syndrome (AIDS), or a fall in CD4 count to $<200/mm^3$.

Effect of HIV on pregnancy

There is some evidence for an association between HIV (especially if advanced) and an increased risk of:

- Miscarriage
- Preterm delivery
- IUGR/low birthweight.

The rate of congenital abnormalities is not increased, although few data are available for HAART.

- In the UK, Europe and USA, asymptomatic HIV infection probably does not increase perinatal mortality, but in developing countries there is evidence of an increased risk.
- Data from Africa suggest a detrimental effect of HIV infection on birthweight, preterm delivery and perinatal mortality.
- The reduction in birthweight is not related to the infant's HIV status, but to the stage of maternal disease.
- The most dramatic effect on pregnancy outcome is related to advanced disease and recurrent infections with poor nutritional status.

Vertical transmission

Rates of vertical transmission without prophylactic therapy vary:

- 15–20% in the UK and Europe.
- 15–30% in the USA.
- 25–40% in sub-Saharan Africa.

Transmission of HIV from mother to child may occur:

- *In utero* (antepartum)
- Through exposure to maternal blood and bodily fluids at the time of delivery (intrapartum)
- By breast-feeding (postpartum).

Two-thirds of vertical transmission seems to occur around delivery, but breast-feeding can double the transmission rate (from 15–30%), especially if maternal infection is acquired postnatally.

The factors that increase the likelihood of vertical transmission are as follows:

- Maternal viral load (most important risk factor)
- Seroconversion (associated with high viral loads) during pregnancy
- Advanced maternal disease
- Poor immunological status (low CD4 counts and low CD4:CD8 ratios)
- Prolonged rupture of membranes (>4 hours)
- Preterm labour
- Vaginal delivery
- Antepartum invasive procedures (amniocentesis, chorionic villous sampling, fetal blood sampling)
- Intrapartum invasive procedures (episiotomy, instrumental delivery and fetal scalp electrodes)
- Prematurity (especially <35 weeks)
- Low birthweight
- Breast-feeding
- Smoking
- Chorioamnionitis
- Intercurrent sexually transmitted diseases
- Vitamin A deficiency
- Unprotected sex with multiple partners
- Use of illicit drugs.

Management

- HIV-positive pregnant women should be jointly followed by an HIV specialist, an obstetrician and a midwife with expertise in managing HIV pregnancy, and a paediatrician.
- Those with CD4 counts <200/mm^3, or those with AIDS and a previous

episode of *Pneumocystis* pneumonia should be given prophylaxis to reduce the risk of *Pneumocystis* pneumonia (see also chapter 4, p. 70) and to protect against *Toxoplasma* reactivation. Co-trimoxazole (Septrin) is the usual drug and the benefits of its use outweigh any theoretical risk of folic acid antagonism. Folate 5 mg should be co-prescribed. Nebulised pentamidine is an alternative agent.

■ Termination of pregnancy should be discussed with women with advanced disease because of the increased risk of vertical transmission, the risk of opportunistic disease, and the reduced life expectancy of the woman.

Antiretroviral therapy

■ The following drug regimens have been shown in randomised clinical trials to decrease vertical transmission of HIV:
  – Zidovudine (azidothymidine, AZT) monotherapy (antepartum, intra-partum, neonatally)
  – AZT/3TC (intrapartum, neonatally)
  – Nevirapaine (intrapartum, neonatally).

■ The potential disadvantages of a policy recommending AZT for all HIV-posit-ive pregnancies include:
  – Expense (particularly relevant for developing countries)
  – The mother may become less sensitive to AZT when she requires it for control of her own disease
  – 80% of babies will be unnecessarily exposed to AZT and its risks (e.g. anaemia).

■ There are no trials completed with HAART regimens, but these result in optimal reductions in viral load and the risk of perinatal transmission is extremely low in women with undetectable plasma viral loads. Very few peri-natal HIV infections have been reported in infants exposed to HAART.

■ AZT prophylaxis (antepartum, intrapartum, neonatally) should be offered to all HIV-positive women. This reduces vertical transmission from 25% to 8%. If in addition delivery is by elective caesarean section and the infant is not breast-fed, perinatal transmission rates are as low as <2%.

■ In women already receiving antiretroviral therapy, AZT should be added or substituted for another nucleoside analogue.

Intrapartum management

■ Elective caesarean section has been shown to reduce perinatal HIV transmis-sion. This is of most benefit in women with high viral loads.

■ There is no evidence that caesarean section reduces vertical transmission if performed after the onset of labour or after rupture of the membranes.

■ HIV-infected women have higher rates of postoperative complications.

- In women receiving HAART or with very low or undetectable viral loads, it is possible that elective caesarean section does not reduce what is already a low transmission risk.

- A blanket policy of caesarean section for all HIV-positive women is not appropriate, but HIV status should be added to the equation when considering mode of delivery for obstetric, medical, and patient preference indications.

- Women should be informed of available data concerning reduction of transmission with elective caesarean section.

- In a study, vaginal cleansing with chlorhexidine only decreased HIV transmission if the membranes had been ruptured for >4 hours before vaginal delivery.

- Gloves, aprons and face protection should be employed during delivery. Early artificial rupture of the membranes, application of fetal scalp electrodes and fetal scalp sampling should be avoided.

Postnatal management

- Early cord clamping and early bathing of the baby may reduce the risk of transmission.

- In the developed world, where mortality from formula feeding is extremely low, women should be strongly advised not to breast-feed. In developing countries, the risks of not breast-feeding may outweigh the risk of transmission of HIV in breast milk.

Human immunodeficiency virus – points to remember

- HIV testing should be freely and easily available both before and during pregnancy. In areas of high prevalence (e.g. London) all women should be offered routine HIV testing in early pregnancy.

- Pregnancy probably does not have a major adverse effect on HIV progression in asymptomatic women.

- Advanced HIV infection may adversely influence pregnancy outcome.

- The risk of vertical transmission varies geographically from 15–40% and is largely due to intrapartum exposure. It is most dependent on maternal viral load, and rare with use of HAART.

- Women should be offered prophylactic AZT therapy to decrease perinatal transmission.

- In the developed world, HIV-positive women should be strongly advised not to breast-feed.

- All babies born to HIV-positive women should be followed up by a paediatrician. Virus culture and PCR are the most reliable techniques for determining infection during the first 2 months of age in non-breast-fed children. Conventional antibody tests cannot be used owing to the persistence of placentally transferred maternal IgG.

Other viral infections in pregnancy

Hepatitis viruses and herpes simplex virus are discussed in chapter 11, p. 200. Varicella zoster is discussed in chapter 4, p. 69.

- The majority of maternal viral infections cause little harm to the fetus. Those that may infect or damage the fetus are shown in Table 15.1.
- Three viruses that may be transmitted to the fetus and cause birth defects are varicella, rubella and CMV.
- Viruses that may increase the rate of miscarriage, stillbirth or perinatal death, or cause neonatal illness and congenital infection include: rubella, CMV, herpes, varicella zoster, hepatitis E, mumps, polio, coxsackie B, parvovirus B19, Japanese encephalitis and Lassa fever.

Listeriosis

Incidence

- This is uncommon but important because of the potentially serious outcome in pregnancy.
- Pregnant women and the immunocompromised are at increased risk.

Clinical features

The mother may be asymptomatic or have a febrile flu-like illness. Features include:

- Headache
- Malaise
- Backache
- Abdominal/loin pain (there may be concomitant urinary tract infection)
- Pharyngitis
- Conjunctivitis
- Diarrhoea.

Maternal infection may be severe and lead to adult respiratory distress syndrome.

Table 15.1 – Viruses that may infect or damage the fetus

Virus	Congenital defects	Other manifestations	Comments	Trimester of risk
Rubella	Ocular defects (cataracts, glaucoma, microphthalmia) Congenital heart defects (patent ductus arteriosus), sensorineural hearing loss, mental retardation	Transient hepatosplenomegaly, jaundice, haemolytic anaemia, thrombocytopenic purpura Diabetes Continuing viraemia	Maternal infection symptomatic in 50–70%. Maculopapular rash, lymphadenopathy, arthritis Incubation 14–21 days Infectivity 7 days before to 7 days after appearance of rash	First trimester (Most fetuses affected) Some risk 13–16 weeks (sensorineuronal deafness) Very little risk after 16 weeks
CMV	Microcephaly, hepatosplenomegaly, jaundice, IUGR, thrombocytopenia, chorioretinitis, intracranial calcification	Psychomotor retardation, sensorineural hearing loss Continuing viraemia	Maternal infection usually subclinical 50–60% of women in UK already immune Risk of fetal damage if mother infected = about 4%	All trimesters Virus detectable in amniotic fluid but most infected fetuses not affected
Varicella	Hypoplasia/aplasia of single limbs with cicatrisation of skin, deafness, psychomotor retardation, ocular abnormalities	20% risk of neonatal varicella infection if mother develops clinical chickenpox 5 days before to 2 days after birth	Incubation 14–21 days Infectivity is from 1 day prior to eruption of the rash to 6 days after the rash disappears	All trimesters Highest risk = 13–20 weeks (2% risk of embryopathy)
Polio	No	Fetal death and neonatal disease	Rare in UK because of routine immunisation	
Coxsackie B	No	Myocarditis, meningoencephalitis, neonatal sepsis	Maternal infection often subclinical May cause aseptic meningitis or Bornholm disease	
Parvo-virus B19	No	Miscarriage, hydrops fetalis and anaemia, fetal death	Maternal infection similar to rubella with rash (erythema infectiosum), arthralgia and fever	

Pathogenesis

- Food-borne infection of *Listeria monocytogenes* in humans is decreased by careful attention to food hygiene.
- Pregnant women should be advised to avoid certain high-risk foods such as unpasteurised dairy products (soft, ripened cheeses) and paté.

Diagnosis

- A high index of suspicion is needed.
- Diagnosis is made by culture of gram-positive bacilli, *L. monocytogenes* in blood, placenta, meconium-stained liquor, or from samples from the neonate.

Effect of listeriosis on pregnancy

- Listeriosis may cause mid-trimester miscarriage and premature labour and meconium.
- If the infant survives, perinatal listeriosis is common and indeed may be the first pointer to maternal infection.
- Transplacental passage of *L. monocytogenes* and congenital listeriosis is also recognised.

Management

Prolonged high doses of parental therapy may be required in maternal and perinatal infections. I.v. ampicillin and gentamicin should be given until 1 week after the fever subsides. Amoxycillin and erythromycin have also been used.

Malaria

Incidence

- Prevalence is high in India, South-East Asia, Africa and South America.
- There are approximately 2000 cases reported in the UK annually to the malaria reference laboratory.
- Most UK cases occur in those who have travelled to or emigrated from malarious areas.
- *Plasmodium falciparum* is responsible for the most severe disease and nearly all mortality due to malaria.
- Pregnant women with little or no immunity, such as those from non-endemic areas, are at increased risk of developing severe disease compared to non-pregnant women. Their maternal and perinatal mortality rates are increased.
- Immunity to malaria is altered by pregnancy. In endemic countries, malaria is a particular problem in primigravidae who have higher rates of parasitaemia. The risk of malaria decreases with successive pregnancies.
- Over 40% of cases of severe anaemia in pregnancy may be prevented by use of effective anti-malarials in pregnant women in endemic areas.

Clinical features

The predominant features are fever, rigors, nausea, abdominal pain and headache. Severe disease in pregnancy includes:

- Hypoglycaemia
- Severe anaemia
- Pulmonary oedema
- Hyperpyrexia
- Cerebral malaria.

Pathogenesis

- Malaria is a protozoan infection caused by *Plasmodium falciparum*, *P. vivax*, *P. malariae* or *P. ovale*.
- Transmission occurs through the bite of an infected female *Anopheles* mosquito.
- In pregnancy, parasites sequester in the placenta, where infection may be very heavy.

Diagnosis

- This is made by detection of parasites on a peripheral blood smear.
- Peripheral parasitaemia >2% should be regarded as severe disease.
- In immune women, peripheral films may be negative despite heavy placental infection.

Effects of malaria on pregnancy

- Malaria increases the risk of second-trimester miscarriage, premature labour and low birthweight. The low birthweight may be due to prematurity or IUGR.
- Malarial parasites may be detected in placentae and congenital malaria can result from transplacental spread or maternal–fetal transmission at parturition.
- Parasites are usually rapidly cleared, probably because the neonate has passive immunity.
- Babies born to non-immune women with untreated or incompletely treated malaria may be severely affected. Parasite clearance should be the aim prior to delivery.

Management

- Pregnant women with malaria should be admitted for treatment because of their increased risk of hypoglycaemia and severe disease.

■ Immune women (i.e. those who have arrived recently from endemic areas) without severe disease may be managed as outpatients. Immigrants from sub-Saharan Africa who have lived in the UK and return intermittently to Africa are likely to be non-immune.

■ Haemoglobin and platelet count should be checked regularly.

■ Blood glucose should be checked initially and 2-hourly when quinine is first commenced.

Antimalarials

■ Prophylaxis and treatment depend on the plasmodium type and the local pattern of drug resistance. Expert advice should always be sought.

■ Chloroquine is the drug of choice for *P. vivax*, *P. malariae*, and *P. ovale*, provided the woman is not ill. Chloroquine is safe for use in pregnancy.

■ Quinine is the drug of choice for *P. falciparum*. There is a particular risk of severe hypoglycaemia. Oral therapy is 10 mg/kg t.d.s. for a minimum of 5 days until clearance of parasitaemia. I.v. therapy is 20 mg/kg over 4 hours followed by 10 mg/kg over 4 hours t.d.s.

■ A single treatment dose of pyrimethamine-sulphadoxine (Fansidar®) is given following parasite clearance. Folate supplementation (10 mg/day) should be given to pregnant women receiving proguanil or pyrimethamine, which are folate antagonists, and these should be avoided in the first trimester.

■ Mefloquine, used for quinine-resistant malaria, has caused teratogenesis in animals and should be avoided.

■ Pregnant women should be discouraged from travelling to malaria-endemic areas. Proguanil and chloroquine are probably the safest drugs used for malarial prophylaxis.

■ Immigrant women resident in the UK wishing to return to a malarial-endemic area should be counselled regarding the likely decline in their immunity.

Further reading

Connor, E.M., Sperling, R.S., Gelber, R. et al. (1994) Reduction of maternal–infant transmission of human immunodeficiency virus type-1 with zidovudine treatment. *N. Engl. J. Med.*, **331**, 1173–1180.

Dorman, E. and Shulman, C. (2001) Malaria in pregnancy. *Curr. Obstet. Gynaecol.*, 10(**4**), 181–189.

Penn, Z.J. and Ahmed, S. (2001) Human immunodeficiency virus in pregnancy. *Curr. Obstet. Gynaecol.*, 10(**4**), 190–195.

Scarlatti, G. (1996) Paediatric HIV infection. *Lancet*, **348**, 863–868.

Drugs to avoid in pregnancy

Absolutely contraindicated	Page reference	Relatively contraindicated	Page reference
Cytotoxic drugs methotrexate cyclophosphamide busulphan	140	**Psychotropic drugs** lithium	
Vitamin A analogues acitretin isotretinoin	242	**Anticoagulant drugs** warfarin	47
Cardiovascular drugs ACE inhibitors, e.g. enalapril angiotensin II inhibitors, e.g. losartan spironolactone	15 127	**Cardiovascular drugs** β-blockers minoxidil **Diuretics** (appropriate to treat pulmonary oedema)	14
Antifungal drugs griseofulvin ketoconazole itraconazole fluconazole terbinafine		**Antibiotics** tetracycline ciprofloxacin aminoglycosides chloramphenicol trimethoprim (first trimester) nitrofurantoin (near term)	69, 183, 185
Antihelminthic drugs mebendazole		**Antileprobic drugs** dapsone (third trimester)	
Anti-inflammatory drugs NSAIDs (late third trimester) COX-2 inhibitors colchicine	137	**Anticonvulsant drugs** phenobarbitone phenytoin sodium valproate carbamazepine	159
Endocrine drugs radioactive iodine sex hormones octreotide	104	**Endocrine drugs** carbimazole propylthiouracil chlorpropamide	97, 102
Other drugs thalidomide mefloquine bisphosphonates misoprostol statins and fibrates tamoxifen nicotine mycophenolate mofetil			
Live vaccines, e.g. MMR, rubella			

ACE: angiotensin-converting enzyme; NSAIDs: non-steroidal anti-inflammatory drugs; COX-2: cyclo-oxygenase type-2-selective.

- For all the drugs listed above, risks must be balanced against potential benefits.
- The teratogenic potential of some of the drugs classified as 'absolutely contraindicated' is sufficiently high to justify termination of a pregnancy following inadvertent exposure, e.g. methotrexate or thalidomide. For others there are theoretical reasons to avoid their use in pregnancy, but they carry a low risk of teratogenesis and therefore there is no justification for termination (e.g. rubella vaccine, simvastatin, ACE inhibitors).
- For the drugs listed as 'relatively contraindicated' there are situations in which their use is appropriate and where no safer alternatives exist, for example warfarin in women with prosthetic heart valves, propylthiouracil in women with thyrotoxicosis, or anti-epileptic drugs.
- β-blockers should be avoided in the treatment of hypertension but may be indicated to control tachyarrhythmias. Diuretics should be avoided in the treatment of hypertension but are appropriate in the treatment of pulmonary oedema.

Normal laboratory values in pregnancy/ non-pregnancy

(This table is also found on the inside back cover)

	Non-pregnant	Pregnant	Trimester		
			1	2	3
Full blood count					
Hb g/dl	12–15	11–14			
WBC × 10^9/l	4–11	6–16			
Platelets × 10^9/l	150–400	150–400			
MCV fL	80–100	80–100			
CRP g/l	0–7	0–7			
Renal function					
Urea mmol/l	2.5–7.5		2.8–4.2	2.5–4.1	2.4–3.8
Creatinine μmol/l	65–101		52–68	44–64	55–73
K mmol/l	3.5–5.0	3.3–4.1			
Na mmol/l	135–145	130–140			
Uric acid mmol/l	0.18–0.35		0.14–0.23	0.14–0.29	0.21–0.38
24-hour protein g	<0.15	<0.3			
24-hour creatinine clearance ml/min	70–140		140–162	139–169	119–139
LFTs					
Bilirubin μmol/l	0–17		4–16	3–13	3–14
Total protein g/l	64–86	48–64			
Albumin g/l	35–46	28–37			
AST iu/l	7–40		10–28	11–29	11–30
ALT iu/l	0–40	6–32			
GGT iu/l	11–50		5–37	5–43	3–41
Alk phosph iu/l	30–130		32–100	43–135	133–418
Bile acids μmol/l	0–14	0–14			
TFTs					
fT4 pmol/l	11–23		11–22	11–19	7–15
fT3 pmol/l	4–9		4–8	4–7	3–5
TSH mu/l	0–4		0–1.6	0.1–1.8	0.7–7.3

ALP: alkaline phosphatase; ALT: alanine aminotransferase; AST: aspartate aminotransferase; GGT: gamma-glutamyl transpeptidase; LFTs: liver function tests; TFTs: thyroid function tests; WBC: white blood cell.

Adapted from: Girling, J.C. (1996) Thyroid disease and pregnancy. *Br. J. Hosp. Med.*, **56,** 316–320.
Girling, J.C., Dow, E. and Smith, J.H. (1997) Liver function tests in pre-eclampsia: importance of comparison with a reference range derived for normal pregnancy. *Br. J. Obstet. Gynaecol.*, **104,** 246–250.
Burrow, G.N. and Ferris, T.F. (1995) *Medical Complications During Pregnancy*, 4th edn. Philadelphia: WB Saunders.

Differential diagnoses of medical problems in pregnancy

Table 1 – Breathlessness

Differential diagnosis	Important clinical features	Investigations
Physiological	Can occur at any stage of pregnancy, but is most common in the last trimester May be most apparent at rest or when speaking	This is a diagnosis of exclusion, which although common should only be made once the diagnoses below have been considered
Anaemia§	May not cause symptoms until severe May be associated with lethargy	Full blood count
Asthma‡	Often associated with cough and/or wheezy breathing Symptoms are usually worse at night and on waking	The diagnosis is usually made on the history PEFR may be normal in clinic If there is doubt about the diagnosis, ask the woman to measure her own PEFR at home (morning and night) and look for diurnal variation and morning 'dipping' Response to inhaled bronchodilators is another confirmatory feature
Pulmonary embolus†	Onset is usually sudden and associated with pleuritic or central (large pulmonary embolus) chest pain Worse on exercise and may be associated with haemoptysis Look for associated sinus tachycardia, raised JVP A high index of suspicion is needed and this diagnosis should always be considered in a pregnant or postpartum woman The risk is higher in obese, older women, post-caesarean section and in those with previous thromboembolism or thrombophilia	ECG (sinus tachycardia, tall peaked p-waves in II) Right heart strain (S_1, Q_3, T_3) may be seen in normal pregnancy) Chest X-ray (often normal but may show pleural effusion, oligaemia, wedge-shaped infarct) Arterial blood gases (hypoxaemia and hypocapnia) The diagnosis should be confirmed with a V/Q lung scan

Cardiac causes There are many cardiac causes of breathlessness; most are uncommon and only two are discussed here	Consider in immigrant women who have never seen a doctor before Breathlessness is due to pulmonary oedema Women may have been asymptomatic at the beginning of pregnancy Ask about orthopnoea, paroxysmal nocturnal dyspnoea and haemoptysis The mid-diastolic murmur may be difficult to hear Look for associated sinus tachycardia	ECG Echocardiogram Chest X-ray
Mitral stenosis*	Pulmonary oedema in association with mitral stenosis is a particular risk immediately following delivery	ECG Echocardiogram Chest X-ray
Peripartum cardiomyopathy*	Most common in the first month after delivery, but can present antenatally More common in older multiparous black women and with multiple pregnancy, pre-eclampsia or hypertension Symptoms and signs of biventricular failure, i.e. tachycardia, pulmonary oedema, peripheral oedema	ECG Echocardiogram Chest X-ray
Pneumonia‡	Often, but not invariably, associated with productive cough and fever Do not forget atypical and viral (particularly chickenpox) pneumonia	Chest X-ray Sputum culture (include AAFB for TB) Full blood count and blood culture Serology (acute and convalescent titres) for atypical pneumonia Cold agglutinins (mycoplasma)
Pneumothorax	Consider if there is sudden onset of pleuritic pain and breathlessness immediately following spontaneous vaginal delivery Look for surgical emphysema	Chest X-ray
Hyperventilation/anxiety	May be associated with paraesthesiae of hands or around mouth	Arterial blood gases show hypocapnia without hypoxaemia

*See also chapter 2; †see also chapter 3; ‡see also chapter 4; §see also chapter 14. AAFB: acid + alcohol-fast bacilli; ECG: electrocardiogram; JVP: jugular venous pressure; PEFR: peak expiratory flow rate; TB: tuberculosis; V/Q: ventilation/perfusion.

Table 2 – Palpitations

Differential diagnosis	Important clinical features	Investigations
Physiological*	Some pregnant women are more aware of their heart beating due to the increased cardiac output May be most apparent at rest, especially when lying down	None
Ectopic beats	Atrial and ventricular premature beats are common in pregnancy, but have no adverse effects on the mother or fetus Close questioning may reveal the palpitations to be due to a 'thumping' sensation. This results from the large cardiac output associated with a beat that follows a long compensatory diastolic pause following a ventricular premature conducted beat More common at rest	ECG
Sinus tachycardia	An increase in heart rate of 10–20 b.p.m. is part of the physiological adaptation to pregnancy Women may be aware of a sinus tachycardia that is appropriate, for example following exercise Although a sinus tachycardia may be a feature of normal pregnancy, it requires selective investigation to exclude respiratory (e.g. asthma, pulmonary embolism) or cardiac (e.g. mitral stenosis, peripartum cardiomyopathy) pathology and hypovolaemia, bleeding or sepsis, or any of the following causes	ECG Thyroid function tests Full blood count Arterial blood gases Echocardiogram

Supraventricular tachycardia†	Paroxysmal SVT is the commonest arrhythmia encountered in pregnancy. It usually pre-dates the pregnancy but may become more frequent in pregnancy It may be due to pre-excitation from accessory pathways such as in Wolff–Parkinson–White syndrome	ECG Holter monitor (24-hour tape) Thyroid function tests Echocardiogram
Thyrotoxicosis‡	All cases of documented sinus tachycardia, SVT, or atrial fibrillation or flutter should have thyroid function measured	ECG Thyroid function tests (include free T4)
Phaeochromocytoma§	This is rare but dangerous and therefore should be considered in cases where there is associated hypertension, headache, sweating or anxiety Attacks may occur while the patient is in the supine position	24-hour urinary catecholamines Ultrasound of adrenals

*See pp 22 and 24; †see p. 38; ‡see p. 101. §see p. 128. ECG: electrocardiogram; SVT: supraventricular tachycardia.

Table 3 – Chest pain

Differential diagnosis	Important clinical features	Investigations
Musculoskeletal	Pain may be related to movement of the arms and torso There may be localised chest wall tenderness Infection with coxsackie B virus (Bornholm disease) may cause chest wall pain due to involvement of the intercostal muscles	None
Gastro-oesophageal reflux*	Pain may be related to eating and is often worse at night due to the recumbent position Pain is usually retrosternal, 'sharp', 'burning', and may be associated with waterbrash and regurgitation or vomiting Symptoms are generally worse in later pregnancy Pain often responds to antacid medication	None
Pulmonary embolism†	Pain may be pleuritic in nature, except with massive pulmonary embolism, causing central chest pain Onset is usually sudden and associated with breathlessness. There may be associated haemoptysis Look for sinus tachycardia and a raised jugular venous pressure A high index of suspicion is needed and this diagnosis should always be considered in a pregnant or postpartum woman with breathlessness and/or chest pain The risk is higher in obese, older women, post-caesarean section and in those with previous thromboembolism or thrombophilia	Chest X-ray ECG Arterial blood gases Lung scan
Pneumonia/pleurisy‡	Pain is usually pleuritic There may be associated fever, cough, sputum or breathlessness Bacterial infections are usually associated with a raised white cell count	Chest X-ray Sputum culture White cell count
Pneumothorax	Pain is pleuritic and associated with breathlessness Consider if there is sudden onset of pleuritic pain and breathlessness immediately following spontaneous vaginal delivery Look for surgical emphysema	Chest X-ray

Ischaemic/cardiac causes§	Pain is usually central and 'crushing' with radiation to the neck or left arm Pain is usually worse on, or precipitated by, exercise Ischaemic heart disease is more common in smokers	ECG Chest X-ray
Aortic dissection‖	Pain is severe and may radiate to the back There may be symptoms or signs from territory supplied by the coronary, carotid, subclavian, spinal or common iliac arteries, or aortic regurgitation	Chest X-ray Chest CT Chest MRI

*See p. 228; †see chapter 3; ‡see chapter 4; §see p. 36. ‖p. 37. CT: computerised tomography; ECG: electrocardiogram; MRI: magnetic resonance imaging.

Table 4 – Heart murmur (see also chapter 2)

Differential diagnosis	Important clinical features	Investigations
Physiological	There is an isolated ESM present in up to 95% of pregnant women It is caused by turbulence related to the increased blood volume and cardiac output of pregnancy The murmur may be audible all over the praecordium and into the neck, and sometimes even in the interscapular area Women with an ESM caused by pregnancy do not have a heart murmur when they are not pregnant and this may be ascertained from a careful history of previous medical check-ups	None
Flow murmur	These are also usually ejection systolic murmurs often loudest over the pulmonary area They are present outside of pregnancy but are also innocent Many women have been previously investigated and require no further investigation in pregnancy The differentiation between flow murmurs confined to pregnancy and those present outside pregnancy is not important	None
Structural defect	Auscultatory pointers to a structural lesion include: – a pan-systolic murmur (suggesting a ventricular septal defect or mitral or tricuspid regurgitation – late systolic murmurs (suggesting mitral valve prolapse) – ESM associated with a palpable thrill, additional heart sounds (other than a third heart sound, which is also common in pregnancy), e.g. ejection click of aortic or pulmonary stenosis or opening snap of mitral stenosis – very loud systolic murmurs – any diastolic murmur (requires further investigation with echocardiography) A high index of suspicion with a lower threshold for echocardiography is required in recent immigrants, especially from areas with a high incidence of rheumatic fever, who may never have seen a doctor or been examined prior to pregnancy	Echocardiogram ECG

ECG: electrocardiogram; ESM: ejection systolic murmur.

Table 5 – Hypertension

Differential diagnosis	Important clinical features	Investigations
'White-coat hypertension'	Hypertension only evident when readings are taken by medical/nursing/midwifery staff Often worse in hospital Does not usually settle completely with repeated readings in hospital setting	Home blood-pressure monitoring Ambulatory blood-pressure recording
Essential hypertension*	Hypertension pre-dates the pregnancy or is discovered in early pregnancy A positive family history is common Pre-eclampsia or pregnancy-induced hypertension may be superimposed More common in Afro-Caribbean and older women	Urea + electrolytes + creatinine Urinalysis Appropriate investigations as below to exclude the following conditions
Pregnancy-induced hypertension*	Usually develops after 20 weeks' gestation No associated features of pre-eclampsia Usually settles within 6 weeks postpartum Often recurs in subsequent pregnancies	Urinalysis Full blood count Urea + electrolytes + creatinine Uric acid and liver function tests Ultrasound scan of fetus
Pre-eclampsia*	Usually develops after 20 weeks' gestation Associated features include: proteinuria, hyperuricaemia, thrombocytopenia, raised transaminases, intrauterine growth restriction, eclampsia, renal impairment Usually settles within 6 weeks postpartum	Urinalysis Full blood count and coagulation screen if platelets <100 × 10⁹/l Urea + electrolytes + creatinine Uric acid and liver function tests Ultrasound scan of fetus

Table 5 – *continued*

Differential diagnosis	Important clinical features	Investigations
Renal hypertension§	Hypertension associated with renal disease, for example reflux nephropathy, diabetes, glomerulonephritis, polycystic kidney disease, renal artery stenosis May be associated with proteinuria, haematuria, renal impairment, active urinary sediment	Urea + electrolytes + creatinine Urinalysis and microscopy Creatinine clearance 24-hour urinary protein Renal ultrasound
Cardiac hypertension† **Co-arctation of the aorta**	Radiofemoral delay or weak femoral pulses may suggest co-arctation of the aorta	Echocardiogram Chest X-ray
Cushing's syndrome‡	Hypertension may be associated with excessive weight gain, extensive purple striae, diabetes or impaired glucose intolerance, easy bruising, hirsutism, acne or proximal myopathy	ACTH Cortisol High-dose dexamethasone-suppression test US, CT or MRI of the adrenals CT or MRI of the pituitary
Conn's syndrome‡	Hypokalaemia (serum potassium <3.0 mmol/l)	Urea + electrolytes + creatinine Plasma renin Plasma aldosterone US, CT or MRI of the adrenals
Phaeochromocytoma†	Hypertension may be sustained or labile, occurring in paroxysms associated with palpitations, anxiety, sweating, headache, vomiting or glucose intolerance	24-hour urinary catecholamines US, CT or MRI of the adrenals

*See also chapter 1; †see also chapter 2; ‡see also chapter 7; §see also chapter 10. ACTH: adrenocorticotrophic hormone; CT: computerised tomography; MRI: magnetic resonance imaging; US: ultrasound.

Table 6 – Abnormal thyroid function tests*

Pattern of abnormality versus normal non-pregnant ranges in women	Possible diagnoses	Comments/further investigation
↑ Total T4 ↑ Total T3 Normal free T4 Normal TSH	Normal in pregnancy	
↓ Free T4 (mild) ↑ TSH (mild)	Normal in third trimester Mild hypothyroidism	Refer to normal ranges for third trimester (Appendix 2) Check thyroid autoantibodies
Normal free T4 ↑ TSH	May be normal feature in first trimester May represent 'compensated' hypothyroidism Treated hypothyroidism possibly with a poorly compliant patient	Repeat thyroid function tests in second trimester Check thyroid autoantibodies TSH may remain high in the initial phases of treatment of hypothyroidism
↑ Free T4 ↓ TSH	May be associated with hyperemesis In the absence of nausea or vomiting, or in association with other symptoms preceding pregnancy, this suggests thyrotoxicosis	Does not require treatment if due to hyperemesis Abnormality resolves with improvement in hyperemesis Check thyroid-stimulating antibodies to help confirm diagnosis of thyrotoxicosis and assess risk of fetal hyperthyroidism
↓ TSH ↓ Free T4	Secondary (pituitary failure) or tertiary (hypothalamic failure), hypothyroidism or non-thyroidal illness	Secondary and tertiary hypothyroidism are both rare
Normal free T4 ↓ TSH	Treated thyrotoxicosis, possibly with an intermittently compliant patient May be a normal feature in first trimester	TSH remains suppressed in the initial phases of treatment of hyperthyroidism Repeat thyroid function tests in second trimester

*See also chapter 6 and Appendix 2. T3: tri-odothyronine; T4: thyroxine; TSH: thyroid-stimulating hormone.

Table 7 – Headache

Differential diagnosis	Important clinical features	Investigations
Tension headache‡	Often related to periods of stress and may occur daily Features of migraine are usually absent	
Migraine‡	Headache is often throbbing, unilateral Prodomal symptoms, usually visual, include: scotoma, teichopsia, fortification spectra Nausea, vomiting, photophobia Transient hemianopia, aphasia, sensory symptoms or hemiplegia may occur but there are no residual physical signs following the attack	
Drug-related headache	Use of vasodilators and calcium antagonists in particular	
Epidural-related headache	Headache is often frontal and postural (relieved by lying down) Commonly associated with dural tap May be associated with neck stiffness, tinnitus, visual symptoms and rarely seizures Onset is usually within 24 hours after siting epidural block	
Hypertension/pre-eclampsia*	May be severe and associated with flashing lights	Urinalysis Full blood count and coagulation screen if platelets $<100 \times 10^9$/l Urea + electrolytes + creatinine Uric acid and liver function tests
Benign intracranial hypertension‡	Headache is often retro-orbital More common in obesity Associated with diplopia, papilloedema Cerebrospinal fluid pressure is increased	CT or MRI Lumbar puncture

Subarachnoid haemorrhage‡	Headache is usually sudden and severe, often occipital Associated vomiting, neck stiffness, loss of (or impaired) consciousness, sudden collapse Papilloedema Focal neurological signs are often, but not invariably, present	CT or MRI Magnetic resonance angiography
CVT†	Usually occurs postpartum Associated with seizures, vomiting, photophobia, impaired consciousness and signs of raised intracranial pressure 30–60% of patients have focal signs that may be transient, such as hemiparesis CVT may cause fever and leukocytosis	CT or MRI Venous angiography MRI Thrombophilia screen
Meningitis	Features include: malaise, fever, rigors, photophobia, vomiting and neck stiffness Petechial rash suggests meningococcal infection	Blood cultures CT to exclude raised intracranial pressure prior to lumbar puncture
Space-occupying lesion	Headache may be focal Onset is usually gradual and may be associated with progressive localising signs and/or seizures	CT or MRI

*See also chapter 1; † see also chapter 3; ‡see also chapter 9. CVT: cerebral vein thrombosis; CT: computerised tomography; MRI: magnetic resonance imaging.

Table 8 – Convulsions

Differential diagnosis	Important clinical features	Investigations
Idiopathic epilepsy§	Usually a preceding history, but idiopathic epilepsy may occasionally present for the first time in pregnancy	Seizures occurring for the first time in pregnancy should be investigated with CT or MRI and EEG
Secondary epilepsy Due to previous surgery, intracranial mass lesions, antiphospholipid syndrome‡	APS may be associated with a history of thromboembolism, fetal loss or thrombocytopenia	Anticardiolipin antibodies Lupus anticoagulant
Eclampsia*	Features of pre-eclampsia may be mild or delayed	Blood pressure Urinalysis Full blood count and coagulation screen if platelets $<100 \times 10^9/l$ Urea + electrolytes + creatinine Uric acid and liver function tests
CVT†	Usually occurs postpartum Associated with headache, vomiting, photophobia, impaired consciousness and signs of raised intracranial pressure 30–60% of patients have focal signs that may be transient, such as hemiparesis CVT may cause fever and leukocytosis	CT or MRI Venous angiography MRI Thrombophilia screen
TTP‖	The clinical features may be confused with pre-eclampsia, but hypertension is not common in TTP Most common in the immediate postnatal period Features may include headache, irritability, drowsiness, coma, fever and renal impairment There is microangiopathic haemolytic anaemia	Full blood count and examination of blood film Coagulopathy is not a feature vWF-cleaving protease (metalloprotease) levels are reduced

Condition	Features	Investigations
Ischaemic cerebral infarction or haemorrhagic stroke§	Strokes are most common in the first week after delivery Most ischaemic strokes associated with pregnancy are in the distribution of the carotid and middle cerebral arteries	CT or MRI Echocardiogram (embolic stoke) Antiphospholipid antibodies
Postdural puncture	Preceded by typical postural headache (relieved by lying down) Associated neck stiffness, tinnitus, visual symptoms Onset usually within 4–7 days after dural puncture	
Drug or alcohol withdrawal	History from relatives/friends Precipitated by admission to hospital	Urine and blood toxicology screen
Metabolic causes: – Hypoglycaemia – Hypocalcaemia – Hyponatraemia	Diabetes, hypoadrenalism, hypopituitarism, liver failure Magnesium sulphate therapy, hypoparathyroidism Hyperemesis	Blood glucose Liver function tests and serum calcium Urea + electrolytes
Pseudoepilepsy§ These patients usually have true epilepsy as well	Useful distinguishing features to differentiate 'pseudo fits' include: – Prolonged/repeated seizures without cyanosis – Resistance to passive eye opening – Down-going plantar reflexes – Persistence of a positive conjunctival reflex	EEG/video telemetry

*See chapter 1; †see chapter 3; ‡see chapter 8; §see chapter 9; ‖see chapter 14. CT: computerised tomography; CVT: cerebral vein thrombosis; EEG: electroencephalogram; MRI: magnetic resonance imaging; TTP: thrombotic thrombocytopenic purpura.

Table 9 – Dizziness

Differential diagnosis	Important clinical features	Investigations
Postural hypotension	Related to prolonged standing, or standing from sitting or lying position Side effect of methyldopa therapy	Lying and standing blood pressure
Supine hypotension	Occurs late in the second and third trimesters when lying in the supine position Owing to pressure of the gravid uterus on the inferior vena cava Relieved by assuming the lateral position	
Labyrinthitis	Vertigo and nystagmus may be reproduced by movement of the head, and particularly moving from a sitting to supine position with the head turned to one side May be associated with vomiting	
Cardiac causes:* – Arrhythmia – Aortic stenosis – Hypertrophic cardiomyopathy	May be associated with palpitations, chest pain, breathlessness, or loss of consciousness	ECG Holter monitor (24-hour tape) Echocardiogram

*See also chapter 2. ECG: electrocardiogram.

Table 10 – Collapse

Differential diagnosis	Important clinical features	Investigations
Pulmonary embolus*	Massive pulmonary embolism causing collapse may be associated with central chest pain Onset is usually sudden and associated with breathlessness May be associated with haemoptysis, sinus tachycardia, a raised JVP and signs of right heart strain The risk is higher in obese, older women, post-caesarean section and in those with previous thromboembolism or thrombophilia	Chest X-ray ECG Arterial blood gases Ventilation/perfusion lung scan Pulmonary angiography
Amniotic fluid embolus	Typically occurs during or immediately following a precipitous labour with an intact amniotic sac. Predisposing factors include increasing age, hypertonic uterine contractions, uterine stimulants, uterine trauma and induced labour There is profound shock, respiratory distress and cyanosis Severe postpartum bleeding usually follows due to the associated disseminated intravascular coagulopathy	Chest X-ray (shows pulmonary oedema in the absence of any clinical evidence of left ventricular failure) Coagulation studies
Seizure/eclampsia†	Tonic–clonic seizure is usually followed by post-ictal drowsiness	See Table 8 for differential diagnosis of seizure
Haemorrhage *Obstetric*, e.g. – Placental abruption – Postpartum haemorrhage *Non-obstetric*, e.g. – Ruptured congenital aneurysm	Haemorrhage may be partially or totally concealed May be associated with disseminated intravascular coagulopathy	Full blood count Coagulation studies Fibrinogen Fibrin-degradation products

Table 10 – *continued*

Differential diagnosis	Important clinical features	Investigations
Ruptured ectopic pregnancy	Presents 4–8 weeks from last menstrual period Associated with pelvic pain and possibly vaginal bleeding	Pelvic ultrasound
Subarachnoid haemorrhage[+]	Collapse may be preceded by severe, often occipital, headache of sudden onset Associated vomiting, neck stiffness, loss of (or impaired) consciousness Papilloedema Focal neurological signs are often, but not invariably, present	CT or MRI Magnetic resonance angiography
Cerebral haemorrhage or infarction[+]	Intracerebral haemorrhage may occur in the setting of pre-eclampsia/eclampsia and most cases occur postpartum, although those associated with arteriovenous malformations may present antenatally Most ischaemic strokes associated with pregnancy are in the distribution of the caroid and middle cerebral arteries, and occur in the first week after delivery	CT or MRI
CVT	Usually occurs postpartum Associated with headache, vomiting, seizures, photophobia, impaired consciousness and signs of raised intracranial pressure 30–60% of patients have focal signs such as hemiparesis, which may be transient CVT may cause fever and leukocytosis	CT or MRI Venous angiography MRI Thrombophilia screen
Metabolic causes§		

*See chapter 3; †see chapter 1; ‡see chapter 9; §See Table 8. CT: computerised tomography; CVT: cerebral vein thrombosis; ECG: electrocardiogram; JVP: jugular venous pressure; MRI: magnetic resonance imaging.

Differential diagnosis	Important clinical features	Investigations
Neuropathy (the presentation and causes of polyneuropathies and peripheral neuropathies, for example, diabetes, B12 deficiency, Guillain–Barré syndrome, are no different in pregnancy)	Numbness in distribution of particular nerve or nerve roots, e.g. **Median nerve** (carpal tunnel syndrome) Numbness affects the middle and index fingers and the thumb and may be associated with pain radiating up the forearm. Symptoms are often bilateral and worse at night **Facial nerve** (Bell's palsy; see chapter 9, p. 178) **Lateral cutaneous nerve of the thigh** (meralgia paraesthetica) Commonly presents in the third trimester **Lumbosacral trunk** (especially L4 and L5) Presents postpartum with unilateral foot drop and numbness and/or pain in the distribution of the affected nerve roots More common with large babies, Keilland's forceps delivery, and cephalopelvic disproportion	Electrophysiological studies
Migraine*	Sensory symptoms are usually transient and associated with unilateral headache, nausea, vomiting and photophobia	
Transient ischaemic attacks	Headache usually absent Attacks last minutes to hours, but always <24 hours A search should be undertaken for a possible embolic source (for example, atrial fibrillation)	Carotid Doppler imaging ECG Echocardiogram
Hyperventilation	Associated with anxiety and panic attacks Numbness in the hands and feet, and peri-oral. May be associated with carpopedal spasm, sweating and dizziness	
Multiple sclerosis*	Patient is usually aware of the diagnosis prior to pregnancy, but relapse involving new symptoms may occur in pregnancy or more commonly postpartum	MRI

*See chapter 9. ECG: electrocardiogram; MRI: magnetic resonance imaging.

Table 12 – Proteinuria

Differential diagnosis	Important clinical features	Investigations
Physiological	Trace or 1+ protein only on dipstick testing may represent <0.3 g/24 hours Trace may be ignored. 1+ protein on urinalysis requires further investigation	MSU and 24-hour protein excretion if ≥1+ on dipstick
Urinary tract infection†	May be associated with symptoms of cystitis or pyelonephritis or be asymptomatic Urine microscopy reveals white cells and possibly red cells A significant growth of organisms on urine culture More common in hyperemesis, diabetes, underlying renal disease, postbladder catheterisation and in those receiving immunosuppressive doses of steroids or azathioprine	Urine microscopy and culture A significant growth is 100 000 organism colonies per ml of urine
Pre-eclampsia*	Usually develops after 20 weeks' gestation Proteinuria is not significant unless >0.3 g/24 hours Associated features include: hypertension, hyperuricaemia, thrombocytopenia, raised transaminases, intrauterine growth restriction, eclampsia, renal impairment Usually, but not invariably, settles within 6 weeks postpartum	Blood pressure 24-hour protein excretion Full blood count and coagulation screen if platelets <100 × 10⁹/l Urea + electrolytes + creatinine Uric acid and liver function tests
Underlying renal disease†	Proteinuria usually evident at booking or prior to 20 weeks' gestation Features of pre-eclampsia may be absent unless there is superimposed pre-eclampsia Associated underlying conditions include: diabetes, reflux nephropathy, glomerulonephritis and systemic lupus erythematosus Urine microscopy may reveal co-existent microscopic haematuria, an 'active sediment' with red cell casts There may be associated renal impairment, hypoalbuminaemia, anaemia early in pregnancy and/or hypertension May only be recognised when proteinuria associated with pre-eclampsia fails to resolve completely postpartum	Urine microscopy 24-hour protein excretion Creatinine clearance Renal ultrasound Renal biopsy (uncommon in pregnancy) ANA/anti-dsDNA Blood glucose Hepatitis B

*See chapter 1; †see chapter 10

Table 13 – Abnormal renal function

Differential diagnosis	Important clinical features	Investigations
Pre-eclampsia/HELLP syndrome*	Usually develops after 20 weeks' gestation Associated features include: hypertension, proteinuria, hyperuricaemia, thrombocytopenia, raised transaminases, intrauterine growth restriction and eclampsia. Oliguria is common and not usually accompanied by renal impairment Renal impairment in pre-eclampsia is usually mild but acute renal failure may develop in 7% of those with HELLP syndrome. Usually, but not invariably, it settles within 6 weeks postpartum May be aggravated or precipitated by NSAIDs	Blood pressure 24-hour protein excretion Full blood count and coagulation screen if platelets $<100 \times 10^9/l$ Urea + electrolytes + creatinine Uric acid and liver function tests
Haemolytic uraemic syndrome‡	The clinical features may be confused with pre-eclampsia, but hypertension is less common in HUS Most common in the immediate postnatal period There is a microangiopathic haemolytic anaemia, fever and thrombocytopenia, which may be severe Cerebral features including headache, irritability, drowsiness, seizures and coma make a diagnosis of TTP	Full blood count and examination of blood film Urea + electrolytes + creatinine vWF-cleaving protease (metalloprotease) levels are normal
Pre-renal failure†	This is most commonly due to blood loss following postpartum haemorrhage or placental abruption, or dehydration secondary to vomiting with or without diarrhoea May be aggravated or precipitated by NSAIDs	Blood pressure Full blood count and coagulation studies if platelets $<100 \times 10^9/l$ Central venous pressure

Table 13 – *continued*

Differential diagnosis	Important clinical features	Investigations
Infection, e.g. septic abortion, puerperal sepsis, rarely acute pyelonephritis	The signs of septic shock may be very similar to those of hypovolaemic shock, and fever and leukocytosis are not always present	Full blood count Blood cultures Mid-stream urine High vaginal swab, wound swab Ultrasound: uterus, abdomen, kidneys
Postrenal failure	This is most commonly due to ureteric damage at caesarean section or obstruction	
Underlying renal disease†	Usually detected preconception or in the first half of pregnancy, when renal function is checked because of hypertension, proteinuria, haematuria or urinary tract infection Features of pre-eclampsia may be superimposed Associated underlying conditions include: hypertension, diabetes, reflux nephropathy, glomerulonephritis and systemic lupus erythematosus Urine microscopy may reveal proteinuria, microscopic haematuria, an 'active sediment' with red cell casts May only be recognised when renal impairment associated with pre-eclampsia fails to resolve completely postpartum	Urine microscopy 24-hour urinary protein excretion Creatinine clearance Renal ultrasound Renal biopsy (uncommon in pregnancy) ANA/anti-dsDNA Blood glucose Hepatitis B

*See chapter 1; †see chapter 10; ‡see chapter 14. ANA: anti-nuclear antibodies; HELLP: Haemolysis, Elevated Liver enzymes and Low Platelets; HUS: haemolytic uraemic syndrome; NSAIDs: non-steroidal anti-inflammatory drugs; TTP: thrombotic thrombocytopenic purpura; vWF: von Willebrand factor.

Table 14 – Pruritus

Differential diagnosis	Important clinical features	Investigations
Physiological	No rash except possibly excoriations Usually affects lower legs Normal liver function tests Presents earlier in pregnancy than obstetric cholestasis	Liver function tests
Liver disease*	No rash except possibly excoriations Associated abnormal liver function tests In some cases of obstetric cholestasis, the only abnormality may be elevated bile acids Women with hepatitis C may develop pruritis for the first time in pregnancy Women with primary biliary cirrhosis or sclerosing cholangitis may experience worsening pruritis in pregnancy	Liver function tests Bile acids Coagulation screen Liver ultrasound Hepatitis serology (including CMV and EBV) Anti-smooth muscle antibodies Anti-mitochondrial antibodies
Skin disease (including drug allergies)†	Obvious rash Normal liver function tests	

*See chapter 11; †see chapter 13. CMV: cytomegalovirus; EBV: Epstein–Barr virus.

Table 15 – Jaundice/abnormal liver function tests†

Differential diagnosis	Important clinical features	Investigations
Obstetric cholestasis†	Severe pruritus (especially palms and soles) with onset usually in third trimester	Liver function tests
	There may be associated dark urine, anorexia and malabsorption of fat (and fat-soluble vitamins, e.g. vitamin K) with steatorrhoea	Bile acids
	Jaundice is rare	Coagulation screen
	Moderate elevation in transaminases, alkaline phosphatase and sometimes gamma glutamyl transpeptidase.	Ultrasound of fetus
	Bile acids are increased	Cardiotocography
	Associated with premature labour, fetal distress, meconium-stained liquor, intrauterine death and postpartum haemorrhage	
Gallstones‡	Usually, but not invariably, associated with pain in the right upper quadrant or epigastrium that may radiate through to the back or to the infrascalpular region	Ultrasound of liver and gall bladder
	Nausea, vomiting and indigestion are common	Blood cultures
	Acute cholecystitis may occur at any time in pregnancy and causes more severe pain than biliary colic	
	There is associated tenderness and guarding in the right hypochondrium	
	There may be fever and shock depending on the severity of the gall bladder sepsis	
Viral hepatitis†	May present at any gestational period	Liver function tests
	There may be a history of foreign travel, but its absence does not exclude the diagnosis	Coagulation screen
	Associated nausea, vomiting, anorexia, fever, malaise and jaundice	Hepatitis serology including CMV and EBV
	Moderate-to-severe elevation in transaminases; raised bilirubin	

Condition	Features	Investigations
Pre-eclampsia/ HELLP syndrome*	Usually develops after 20 weeks' gestation. Associated features include: hypertension, proteinuria, hyperuricaemia, thrombocytopenia, intrauterine growth restriction, eclampsia, renal impairment, and in the case of HELLP syndrome, epigastric or right upper quadrant pain, nausea and vomiting, tenderness in the right upper quadrant and haemolysis	Blood pressure 24-hour protein excretion Full blood count and coagulation screen if platelets $<100 \times 10^9$/l Blood film Urea + electrolytes + creatinine Uric acid and liver function tests
AFLP†	Associated nausea, anorexia, malaise, vomiting and abdominal pain. There are often co-existing features of mild pre-eclampsia, but hypertension and proteinuria are usually mild. Hyperuricaemia is often marked and out of proportion to the severity of pre-eclampsia. Coagulopathy is often a prominent feature. Jaundice usually appears within 2 weeks of the onset of symptoms and there may be ascites. Liver function is more deranged than in HELLP syndrome and the woman may develop fulminant liver failure with hypoglycaemia, hepatic encephalopathy, and renal failure	Blood pressure 24-hour protein excretion Full blood count and coagulation screen Blood film Urea + electrolyte + creatinine Blood glucose Uric acid and liver function tests CT liver Liver biopsy
Hyperemesis gravidarum‡	Onset before 12 weeks' gestation. Abdominal pain is rare, jaundice very rare. Nausea, vomiting, dehydration, profound weight loss, ketonuria. Associated 'biochemical thyrotoxicosis' (see chapter 12). Liver function reverts to normal as hyperemesis improves	Urea + electrolytes Thyroid function tests Liver function tests
Sepsis, e.g. acute cholecystitis, ascending cholangitis, puerperal sepsis	Associated fever, abdominal pain	White blood cell count Blood cultures
Drug-induced hepatotoxicity, e.g. methyldopa, halothane, chlorpromazine		

Table 15 – *continued*

Differential diagnosis	Important clinical features	Investigations
Pre-existing/co-existing liver disease†	These diagnoses are usually made prior to pregnancy	Liver function tests ANA
Autoimmune chronic active hepatitis	CAH may present as acute hepatitis or with signs of chronic liver disease and, in the later stages, cirrhosis. Liver function may be markedly deranged. CAH is associated with antibodies to smooth muscle, antinuclear antibodies, and hypergammaglobulinaemia	Anti-smooth-muscle antibodies
PBC	PBC causes pruritus preceding jaundice and hepatomegaly by a few years A raised alkaline phosphatase may be the only biochemical abnormality	Anti-mitochondrial antibodies (95% positive in primary biliary cirrhosis)
Sclerosing cholangitis	50% of patients with sclerosing cholangitis have IBD, although there is no relationship with the severity of the IBD May be asymptomatic or cause intermittent pruritus, jaundice and abdominal pain	Liver ultrasound Liver biopsy

*See chapter 11; †see chapter 12. AFLP: acute fatty liver of pregnancy; ANA: antinuclear antibody; CAH: chronic active hepatitis, CMV: cytomegalovirus; EBV: Epstein–Barr virus; HELLP: Haemolysis, Elevated Liver enzymes and Low Platelets; IBD: inflammatory bowel disease; PBC: primary biliary cirrhosis.

Table 16 – Vomiting

Differential diagnosis	Important clinical features	Investigations
Physiological	Associated nausea 'Morning sickness' is a misnomer; nausea and vomiting may occur throughout the day Onset before 12 weeks' gestation, commonly 6–7 weeks Usually remits by 12–16 weeks' gestation	
Hyperemesis gravidarum	Onset before 12 weeks' gestation Nausea and vomiting are severe enough to cause marked weight loss, dehydration, and ketonuria May be associated with abnormal thyroid and liver function More common with multiple and molar pregnancy	Urea + electrolytes Liver function tests Thyroid function tests Mid-stream urine
Drug-induced, e.g. iron supplements, antibiotics, ergometrine		
Infection, e.g. urinary tract infection, gastroenteritis, cholecystitis	See abdominal pain, Table 17	Mid-stream urine Stool culture Blood cultures Liver and renal US
Pre-eclampsia/HELLP/AFLP	See abdominal pain, Table 17	
Metabolic causes, e.g. uraemia, hyperglycaemia, hypercalcaemia		Urea + electrolytes Blood glucose Liver function tests and calcium

Note: Most of the non-obstetric causes of abdominal pain (see Table 17) may also present with vomiting. AFLP: acute fatty liver of pregnancy; HELLP: Haemolysis, Elevated Liver enzymes, and Low Platelets; US: ultrasound.

Table 17 – Abdominal pain

Differential diagnosis	Important clinical features	Investigations
OBSTETRIC CAUSES		
Ectopic pregnancy/miscarriage	Presents between 4–12 weeks from last menstrual period Pain is in the lower abdomen or pelvis and there may be associated vaginal bleeding	US of uterus
Labour	Pain is intermittent, associated with tightenings and contractions, shortening of the cervix and engagement of the fetal head	Cardiotocography
Placental abruption	Pain may be mild or severe and associated with uterine irritability More common in pre-existing hypertension and pre-eclampsia Not invariably associated with vaginal bleeding and uterine tenderness Very difficult diagnosis to exclude, especially if there are recurrent episodes The absence of visible retroplacental clot on US does not exclude the diagnosis	US of uterus
Ovarian cysts	Pain is unilateral, intermittent and associated with vomiting Cyst visible on US	US of uterus and ovaries
Uterine fibroids	Pain is constant and localised Area of tenderness on uterus coincides with position of fibroid on US More common in black races	US of uterus
Ligamentous pain	Pain is commonly bilateral, 'sharp', 'stitch-like', short-lived and aggravated by movement	
Pre-eclampsia/ HELLP syndrome*	Pain is often epigastric or in the right upper quadrant and usually develops after 20 weeks' gestation	Blood pressure 24-hour urinary protein excretion

	hyperuricaemia, elevated transaminases, thrombocytopenia, intrauterine growth restriction, eclampsia, renal impairment, and in the case of HELLP syndrome, nausea and vomiting; tenderness in the right upper quadrant and haemolysis	screen if platelets $<100 \times 10^9/l$, blood film Urea, electrolytes + creatinine Uric acid and liver function tests US of liver
AFLP§	Pain is usually in the epigastrium or right upper quadrant and associated with nausea, vomiting, anorexia and malaise There are often co-existing features of mild pre-eclampsia, but hypertension and proteinuria are usually mild Hyperuricaemia is often marked and out of proportion to the severity of pre-eclampsia Coagulopathy is often a prominent feature Jaundice usually appears within 2 weeks of the onset of symptoms and there may be ascites Liver function is more deranged than in HELLP syndrome and the woman may develop fulminant liver failure with hypoglycaemia, hepatic encephalopathy, and renal failure	Blood pressure 24-hour protein excretion Full blood count and coagulation screen Blood film Urea + electrolytes + creatinine Blood glucose Uric acid and liver function tests CT of liver Liver biopsy

NON-OBSTETRIC CAUSES

Constipation

See chapter 12

Infection,
e.g. pyelonephritis,‡
cholecystitis‖ pneumonia†

There may be fever and shock depending on the severity of any sepsis **Pyelonephritis** usually causes loin pain, which may radiate round to the abdomen and down into the groin **Cholecystitis** may cause pain in the right upper quadrant or epigastrium, which may radiate through to the back or infrascalpular region There is associated tenderness and guarding in the right hypochondrium Nausea and vomiting are common in both pyelonephritis and cholecystitis	Mid-stream urine Blood cultures US of kidneys US of liver and gall bladder Chest X-ray

Table 17 – *continued*

Differential diagnosis	Important clinical features	Investigations
	Pneumonia, especially affecting the right lower lobe, may cause right upper quadrant pain	
Appendicitis[ll]	Pain associated with nausea, vomiting and rebound tenderness Pain may not localise to the right iliac fossa, especially in late pregnancy	Full blood count US of abdomen
Pancreatitis[ll]	Most attacks occur in the third trimester Epigastric pain radiating through to the back, with nausea and vomiting	Serum amylase US of gall bladder, liver and upper abdomen
Peptic ulcer[ll]	Epigastric pain that may be relieved by food in the case of duodenal ulcer or aggravated by food in gastric ulcer Pain improves with antacids Associated heartburn, nausea and possibly haematemesis	Gastroscopy
Renal colic	Pain is usually in the loin but may radiate round to the abdomen and down into the groin	US of kidneys
Iliac vein thrombosis	Pain is in the left or right iliac fossa There may be swelling and tenderness of the leg or tenderness over the femoral vein Pyrexia may be evident	Doppler US Venogram
Metabolic, e.g. diabetic ketoacidosis, hypercalcaemia		Urea + electrolytes, blood glucose Liver function tests and calcium

*See chapter 1; †see chapter 4; ‡see chapter 10. §see chapter 11; ‖see chapter 12. AFLP: acute fatty liver of pregnancy; HELLP: Haemolysis, Elevated Liver enzymes

Index